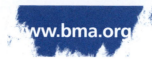

The New GP's Handbook

HOW TO MAKE A SUCCESS OF YOUR EARLY YEARS AS A GP

PETER DAVIES

GP Keighley Road Surgery, Illingworth, Halifax
GP Appraisal Lead, Calderdale PCT
Member, Calderdale Clinical Commissioning Group
Provost, Yorkshire Faculty, RCGP

LINDSAY MORAN

General Practitioner, Leeds
Treasurer and First5® Lead, Yorkshire Faculty of the RCGP

HUSSAIN GANDHI

General Practitioner, Nottingham and Yorkshire Academic Teaching
Fellow, University of Leeds
First5® Lead, Yorkshire Faculty of the RCGP
Owner: www.egplearning.co.uk

with

ADRIAN ROEBUCK

Business Development Manager
SunnyBank Medical Centre, Wyke, Bradford

Foreword by
CLARE J TAYLOR

Chair of Associates in Training Committee, 2008–09
First5®Clinical Lead, 2009–present
Royal College of General Practitioners

Radcliffe Publishing
London • New York

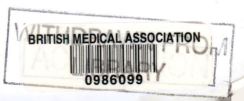

Radcliffe Publishing Ltd
33–41 Dallington Street
London
EC1V 0BB
United Kingdom

www.radcliffepublishing.com

British Library Cataloguing in Publication Data

A catalogue record for this book is available from the British Library.

ISBN-13: 978 184619 594 5

The paper used for the text pages of this book is FSC® certified. FSC (The Forest Stewardship Council®) is an international network to promote responsible management of the world's forests.

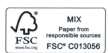

Typeset by Darkriver Design, Auckland, New Zealand
Printed and bound by TJI Digital, Padstow, Cornwall, UK

Contents

Foreword   v

About the authors   vii

Acknowledgements   ix

 1 Introduction   1

 2 The nature of a profession   7

 3 The primary care landscape   13

 4 The work of general practice   29

 5 Levels of medical effectiveness   37

 6 How to find a job   45
    A Partnerships   56
    B Freelance   59
    C Salaried   70

 7 Continuing professional development, appraisal and revalidation   75
    A Your licence to practise   80
    B Continuing professional development   82
    C Appraisal   92
    D Personal development plans   105
    E Revalidation   107
    F Clinical governance   110

 8 Leadership   113

 9 Commissioning   125

10 A day in the life of a GP   139

11 The doctor's bag   143

12 How to stay sane and healthy as a GP   147

13 Dealing with isolation and medical uncertainty   157

14 Adapting consultation skills to the world of actual general
practice   165

15 The business of general practice   173

16 How to handle a complaint   183

17 How to deal with your heart sinking   195

18 Mentorship   199

19 Learning points   203

20 Ongoing learning and support: what's the best way to
achieve this?   215

Index   223

Foreword

Qualifying as a new GP is an exciting but daunting time. The training years are hard work but they are spent with the comfort of having a trainer in the next room and the regularity of the specialty training scheme which provides an opportunity for peer group learning and support. Then, at the end of training, the new GP enters the world of modern general practice; an independent practitioner for the first time. For some, this transition can feel like 'falling off a cliff'. The Associates in Training Committee 2008–09 at the Royal College of General Practitioners recognised this phenomenon and developed the First5® concept as a way for the college to support new GPs from completion of training through the first 5 years of independent practice. The First5® initiative was launched in 2010 and, while this book has been written independently of the Royal College of General Practitioners, we very much welcome the recognition it shows to the needs of new GPs.

Dr Peter Davies is a knowledgeable and innovative GP with many years of clinical experience. Dr Lindsay Moran and Dr Hussain Gandhi are both dynamic and enthusiastic new GPs who have recently experienced the transition from trainee to qualified GP. Together they have a real understanding of the challenges facing new GPs. Adrian Roebuck is a talented business manager for a local practice in Bradford.

This book begins with a fascinating overview of the history of the profession that is vital to understanding the landscape in which new GPs now find themselves working. Perhaps the most pressing issue when the Certificate of Completion of Training finally arrives is to find a job, and the chapter covering the opportunities and pitfalls involved in this process gives valuable advice for any new GP. The importance of staying physically and mentally healthy is a must for any doctor to consider at an early stage in their career and so several chapters are devoted to this important issue. The key skills that research has shown some new GPs feel less confident in – skills such as practice management, leadership, commissioning and advanced consulting skills – are also covered. Finally, the importance of lifelong learning and continuing professional development in the context of appraisal and revalidation are discussed.

General practice is an exciting and rewarding career that provides a host of opportunities for new GPs entering the profession today. Finding the right job, achieving a good work–life balance and developing a culture of lifelong learning are vital, not only for the fulfilment of new GPs themselves but also for the future of the profession. *The New GP's Handbook* will help you achieve these objectives.

Dr Clare J Taylor
Chair of Associates in Training Committee, 2008–09
First5® Clinical Lead, 2009–present
Royal College of General Practitioners
March 2012

About the authors

Peter Davies graduated from Leeds in 1989 and passed his membership examination for the Royal College of General Practitioners (RCGP) and summative assessment in 1995. He became a GP principal at Alison Lea Medical Centre in East Kilbride in 1996. In 2001, he moved back to his home town of Halifax. He worked as a salaried GP in the deprived area of Mixenden, Halifax, from 2001 to 2005, before moving as a partner to Keighley Road Surgery, Illingworth, Halifax, in 2005. He received his fellowship of the RCGP in 2009.

Peter has many roles beyond his partnership – sometimes to the despair of his partners. He is provost of the Yorkshire Faculty of the RCGP, having previously been chair for many years. He represents the Yorkshire Faculty on the RCGP Council. He is appraisal lead for NHS Calderdale and an elected member of the Calderdale Clinical Commissioning Group. He is a prolific and reflective medical author and has published many articles in the *BMJ*, the *British Journal of General Practice* and elsewhere. He represents experience in this team of authors.

He can be contacted on npgdavies@blueyonder.co.uk.

Lindsay Moran passed her membership examination for the Royal College of General Practitioners in 2009. She has worked as a freelance GP and salaried GP in Leeds. She works as a tutor and facilitator at Leeds University. She has presented research and projects annually at Royal College of General Practitioners and WONCA (World Organization of National Colleges, Academies and Academic Associations of General Practitioners/Family Physicians) conferences. She attended the Yorkshire Faculty as a GP trainee before moving to be First5® representative and subsequently being elected treasurer of the faculty. Aside from her GP and academic work, she runs a local Botox business and is the founder of GP Advance (www.gpadvance.com).

She can be contacted on lindsaymoran@doctors.org.uk and Twitter (@lindsmoran).

Hussain Gandhi passed his membership examination for the Royal College of General Practitioners (RCGP) in 2009. He worked as an academic teaching fellow at the University of Leeds, and clinically as a GP at Caritas Group practice in Halifax until March 2012. He is now expanding his career by maintaining links with his teaching work, as well as becoming a partner at Wellspring Surgery in Nottingham.

He joined the Yorkshire Faculty of the RCGP as an Associate in Training representative and has since become an elected member of the faculty board. He is one of the faculty's First5® representatives, and he and Lindsay organised a Yorkshire RCGP First5® study day held in Leeds in June 2011 that led to this book being written. He has presented on various occasions at the annual RCGP conference, regarding, among other things, areas of technology use in practice, and he currently manages successful primary care websites such as: www. yournhs.co.uk and eGP Learning (www.egplearning.co.uk).

He can be contacted on drgandalf@hotmail.co.uk or on Twitter (@drgandalf52).

Adrian Roebuck is Business Development Manager at SunnyBank Medical Centre, Wyke, Bradford. He led the business strategy session for a Yorkshire Royal College of General Practitioners First5® study day organised by Lindsay and Hussain for June 2011, and he has turned his presentation into Chapter 15 of this book.

Acknowledgements

The authors are grateful to many people for health and advice that has gone into this book. Needless to say we are responsible for the final text and any errors in it.

We are grateful to Dr James Parsons and Dr Clare Taylor for the First5® initiative, and to Clare for her foreword.

Peter would like to thank his partners at Keighley Road Surgery – Dr John Chatterjee, Dr Michael Houghton, Dr Kate Barnes and Dr Katherine Simpson for their tolerance, humour and conversation over time. Also for their specific input in reviewing the clinical chapters.

He is grateful to his wife Michelle for ongoing support and allowing him time to write this book.

He would like to thank Dr Jim Rodger, Dr Malcolm Thomas, Dr Cordelia Paterson, Dr Navjeet Dua, Dr Clare Gerrada and Prof Amanda Howe, for reviewing various sections at an early stage of the book's development and suggesting improvements.

He would like to thank Dr Matt Walsh, Dr Alan Brook, Julie Lawreniuk and other colleagues both clinical and managerial at Calderdale Clinical Commissioning Group for helping him learn about commissioning and its intricacies.

He would like to thank Dr Damian Riley, Dr David Geddes, Dr Andy Godden, Dr Mark Purvis, Dr Colin Pollock and Dr Phil Ayres for helping him improve his understanding of appraisal and revalidation. His fellow appraisers in Calderdale Appraisers Group and their administrator Julie Wan-Sai-Cheong have helped him see what needs to be done to bring the ideas into practice locally.

He is grateful to Yorkshire Faculty for giving him the opportunity to teach on the First5® courses and to his two young co-authors for helping keep the book anchored in the needs of new GPs.

Lindsay would like to thank Dr Clare Taylor for being a fantastic motivational lead for all First5® GPs across the country and for her kind support with this book. That of course leads to a thank you to Dr James Parsons, who with Clare has made the First5® initiative possible.

Lindsay would also like to thank all her GP trainers, Dr Jane Petty, Dr Simon Hall and Dr Sarah Hutchinson, who have encouraged and pushed her throughout her training to keep her working hard and achieving more.

She would like to thank the hard work of the TPDs during her GP training – Dr Helen Allcock, Dr Simon Boyle, Dr Katie Houston and Dr Laura Clegg, especially for the support and efforts when working towards the conferences.

She would like to give thanks to Dr Kirsty Balwin for her support as Chair of Faculty and supporting events that helped this book to be possible.

She would like to thank co-authors, and in particular Dr Peter Davies for his inspirational lead, constant motivation and guidance and as described in the mentorship chapter, she would like to thank her wonderful boyfriend and parents too.

All the writings in this book have been made possible from our time spent in the company of many inspirational people.

Hussain would like to thank Dr Andrew Jackson and Dr Pamela Sides as his Educational Supervisors, his Airedale VTS cohort, and Programe Directors: Dr Jim Hodgson, Dr Helen Wilkinson and the late Dr Elizabeth Clements for their support and tutoring during his GP training. Their guidance enabled him to have the confidence and initiative to accomplish so much.

He would like to thank his co-authors Peter, Lindsay and Adrian, with producing a necessity for all new GPs. The Academic Unit of Primary Care at the University of Leeds has provided clarity and educational support, deserving of a special mention.

Last but not least, he would like to thank his wife and parents for their unwavering support and tolerance with his many activities.

Chapter 1

Introduction

Peter Davies and Lindsay Moran

Si jeunesse savoit, si vieillesse pouvoit . . .
(If the young were to know, if the old were still able . . .)

—Henri Estienne

Welcome to *The New GP's Handbook.*

General practice has never been an easy occupation. But at least in the past there were some clear structures and routes for newly qualified GPs to enter. New GPs could expect to join practices as partners and to progress through the ranks and grow in seniority and confidence as they did so. In the better partnerships the young GP would often be informally mentored by one of his or her older colleagues and gradually he or she could learn the practice management and business skills of general practice.

It is no longer like this. The market for new GPs has altered, the range of options is wider, and the way through the labyrinth is far from clear. As a new GP, you are likely to be rather confused and bewildered by the colourful new world you find yourself in. You may well be struggling to recognise the key features of this new world, and you may have little or no idea where you should position yourself in relation to these key features and which route you should take to get there.

This book is written to help with your bewilderment. We hope that by the end of this book we will have helped you to see clearly where you have got to now and where you want to get to in the future and how to get there. Along the way we hope to help you formulate the strategies you will need to use to define your priorities and so decide which jobs to aim for and which to avoid. We will try to map out the landscape of general practice so that you can navigate your way around it, and succeed in knowing and getting what you want from your professional life and how to overcome the hurdles you will inevitably encounter. Two of us, Lindsay Moran and Hussain Gandhi, are new GPs currently in the swamp of career uncertainties and impending appraisals but lightened with opportunities of new jobs, possible portfolio careers and leadership opportunities.

The need for this book became apparent after a number of meetings and discussions with various young GPs in the first 5 years following completion of their training, and the book itself emerges from events we have run in Yorkshire under the First5® banner of the Royal College of General Practitioners (RCGP). From these events it is clear there are many things newly qualified GPs need to know that are not covered on the vocational training scheme (VTS). Alternatively, maybe as a GP registrar you were taught them but you did not appreciate their significance at the time. These things are very rarely clinical issues – indeed, the great strength of the VTS is that you tend to leave it with competent clinical knowledge and good communication and consultation skills. They are topics that tend to be much more practical, managerial and organisational (these are difficult to teach) and which only become sharply relevant when you enter the world beyond the VTS. If we could get GP training extended to 4 or 5 years (as the RCGP argues strongly for) then we could include most of these topics within the curriculum. However, at present we cannot, and this leaves newly qualified GPs with some significant weaknesses – weaknesses that we hope this book will help to remedy.

The GP VTS can be considered as rather like a womb – a protective environment in which a new life (professional identity) can form. The French word 'naïve' describes the property of just being born. The impression we have is that many new GPs are somewhat naïve. Moreover, the term 'competent but not confident' is currently bandied about. After reading this book you won't be naïve and you will be more confident; it is to be hoped that you will have acquired much of the knowledge of the old, yet without losing your youth.

THE BIRTH OF FIRST5®

In this book we will introduce you to how the RCGP was born and how it grew to be the college it is today. The College Council is attended by a group of motivated 'mover and shaker' GPs who regularly attend meetings at the hub in London. They are an elected collection of experienced doctors with the influence to drive the direction of the college's aims.

Initially, young GPs (particularly trainees) were poorly represented on this council. In 2007 the college became responsible for the licensing examination for all new GPs. This was created as the nMRCGP (new Membership of the Royal College of General Practitioners) examination, a long-overdue synthesis of the previously separate exams of 'summative assessment' and MRCGP. With young and new GPs uncomfortable amidst this change with the college voice coming from only older GPs, it was agreed through discussion that the Associates in Training (AiT) Committee be formed. The committee was first formed in November 2007. After a successful beginning the committee was invited to attend College Council meetings. The College Council realised what an asset the voice of young GPs was, and the AiT Committee has continued to grow in strength.

However, when the AiTs came to the end of their training and were no longer sheltered under the trainee umbrella, they thought forlornly, 'well, what happens to us now?' Like years of GPs before them, these AiTs realised that after qualification the world of general practice is a potentially lonely and unsupported one. Three years of training is arguably not nearly enough training time to be a fully competent solo practitioner generalist of all the specialties. With those GPs who chose to work as salaried doctors or partners, there is hopefully the support of the more experienced GPs at the practice. However, for locums and salaried GPs, especially those who move to new areas, being a GP can be very isolated. Also, young GPs are often desperate not to appear inadequate in their skills; although they know to ask for help when they need it, I (Lindsay) know from conversations with my own peers that this is something you do not wish to do too often. You do not want to look like a fool in front of all the other clever, more experienced doctors when you barely feel like one yourself. Young GPs are a particularly vulnerable group, 'a lost tribe', who are currently more in need of support than any other group. AiTs have good support from the RCGP, their local deaneries and training schemes, but all this disappears on qualification. Equally, and often as a consequence of this, many young GPs see no advantage in continuing their membership with the college.

And so it was that these ex-AiTs sat in a room and saw a blind spot on the GP roller coaster. With the introduction of revalidation it seemed common sense to focus on this new group of GPs, supporting them from qualification until revalidation at 5 years.

Dr James Parsons, an AiT in Sheffield at the time, was the first to describe the concept of First5®. Together with Dr Clare Taylor (the first AiT Committee chair), Dr Parsons formed the First5® group in 2007, the aim of which is to give identity to and to support all newly qualified doctors within the first 5 years post completion of the VTS and the nMRCGP exam. First5® leads were established throughout the country to work on five key pillars:

1. **Connecting**: promoting a sense of belonging and appropriate representation for the First5® cohort within the college. Locally, young GPs are now involved on all faculty boards across the UK to champion the First5® cause.
2. **Networks**: encouraging peer support and mentoring through the development of local networks.

3. **Career mentorship**: highlighting the opportunities a career in general practice offers and helping new GPs get the most out of being a GP.
4. **Continuing professional development (CPD)**: identifying the CPD needs of those within the first 5 years following award of the Certificate of Completion of Training, highlighting existing relevant provision and developing new materials where gaps exist.
5. **Revalidation**: offering support through revalidation for those in the first 5 years following award of the Certificate of Completion of Training.

Although the First5® initiative is only in its early stages, it has now extended to all areas of the UK. It is recognised that there are different needs in the different areas of the country, but just as the AiT Committee grew from a small seed into a successful entity so too has First5®. The RCGP as a college enthusiastically supports this initiative as a service to its newer and younger members. As the authors of this book, we hope *The New GP's Handbook* will help new GPs with these objectives.

The term First5® has become a college trademark, so to avoid infringing this trademark in *The New GP's Handbook* we use the term 'new GPs'; however, when writing this book we were thinking about the specific information needs of GPs in their first 5 years of independent practice after passing the MRCGP examination. We hope new GPs will find this book helpful and that they will be able to use the knowledge and perspectives herein to benefit themselves, enabling them to enjoy their career more and to help their patients better.

HOW THIS BOOK CAME ABOUT

This book came about after a Yorkshire RCGP First5® study day held in Leeds in June 2011. Peter Davies had run a similar session a year earlier with James Parsons ('101 things they didn't teach you on the VTS'). Lindsay Moran and Hussain Gandhi were the two First5® leads on the Yorkshire Faculty Board and had arranged the day and its agenda. Lindsay and Hussain asked Peter, as former chair of the Yorkshire RCGP Faculty to be one of the speakers.

Peter had the chance to listen to the topics and the questions and he realised there was a need to capture the questions and their answers and make them widely available to new GPs. Lindsay and Hussain quickly agreed that this would be a useful project, and the result is *The New GP's Handbook*.

Peter is responsible for writing most of the book. Lindsay has written about the practicalities of life for a new GP, focusing on the hurdles that new GPs need to overcome. Hussain has aided with the above and included his own viewpoints throughout the book, in addition to the editing. Adrian Roebuck led the business strategy session for the aforementioned Yorkshire RCGP First5® study day in June 2011 and has turned his presentation into Chapter 15 of this book. Each chapter begins with the contributing author.

Throughout the process of writing the book, Lindsay and Hussain kept prodding Peter to remind him that once you know something it can sometimes be very difficult to remember that you didn't always know it. The result should be a useful text that is sufficiently down to earth to answer basic questions, and sufficiently elevated to let you understand what is happening, why things are as they are, and how these things may develop in the future. We hope this book inspires you to want to be part of shaping the future of primary care services in the UK.

Some of the topics covered are new, controversial or, indeed, not fully worked out yet by young or by old. In this book we have presented our best current understanding of revalidation, leadership and commissioning, but the information and our views on these topics may change over time. Many experienced GPs may find our accounts of these developments a useful current overview.

Some of the topics are perennials in general practice and are probably existential to our work. We have covered these topics because all GPs, new and old, need strategies for them. Obviously, new GPs cannot have as much experience as their older colleagues. We hope that what is presented here in *The New GP's Handbook* is a useful distillation of the knowledge of older GPs and that this will speed up the learning for newer GPs.

This book is a combination of youth and experience. Our hope as authors is that this book will help to make your first 5 years – and indeed beyond – in general practice more understandable, productive and enjoyable.

REFERENCES

1 Taylor CJ, Parsons J, Sparrow N, *et al.* The first5 concept. *Br J Gen Pract.* 2011; **61**(582): 72–3.
2 Taylor CJ. From the . . . new GP: first5. *InnovAiT.* 2010; **3**(10): 587.

Chapter **2**

The nature of a profession

Peter Davies

If you think it's expensive to hire a professional to do the job, wait until you hire an amateur.

—Red Adair

WHAT IS A PROFESSION?

What is a profession? What does it mean to be a professional? What distinguishes a professional from an amateur? These are all questions worth thinking about as a new GP.[1] You may already have some answers to these questions – you became a member of the profession with your medical degree and your full General Medical Council registration. You are now stepping up, becoming a new member of an important specialty within the profession of medicine. What does this mean to you? What does this mean to others?

A profession arises when any trade or occupation transforms itself through 'the development of formal qualifications based upon education, apprenticeship, and examinations, the emergence of regulatory bodies with powers to admit and discipline members, and some degree of monopoly rights.'[2]

There is often an element of vocation to professions – you are called to them. There is often an element of mission to professions – you are sent out to do something, and that something is usually a noble purpose of some sort that will affect other people and their lives significantly. To some extent, professions are intrusive enterprises: think of divinity and its care for souls, of law and its care for disputes and legal boundaries of behaviour, of doctors and our permission to intrude into the hidden spaces of people's lives and bodies. These are all intensely personal services that need to be provided with great concern for those we treat;

they require deep knowledge and specific standards of behaviour if they are to be done well or even at all. These standards of knowledge and behaviour and their focus on providing services to others are what mark out a profession from an ordinary job. This is not to say that people in ordinary jobs cannot do a good job, or indeed provide very valuable services, or even be very professional about how they go about their work. However, in a profession we should start from such high standards as the basic, and be looking to achieve and contribute even more. As such, senior professionals acquire a significant burden of duties and obligations, and gain status to the extent that they live up to these and deliver them well. As a new GP you may be coming to realise some of the burden we carry as professionals and be looking to find ways of owning this burden, rather than finding it too burdensome. We hope this book will help you with these tasks.

Being a professional brings status and significant reward, both personal and financial. However, it also brings significant hassles and significant responsibilities. Becoming a professional takes a lot of training, and once you are set up in a profession it is a wrench to move to another. The more you speak with professionals from other fields, the more you realise that although their core skill – accountancy, law and so forth – is different to yours, the basic stresses and hassles are actually very similar.

People can view professions in differing ways: some emphasise the character and nobility of the profession and the greatness of its cause; others view professionals as over-trained tradesmen who could do with being brought down a peg or two. In the following section we look at what the economists make of professions. Ultimately, all activity in terms of jobs and services has an economic basis; being a professional and maintaining a profession's distinctiveness (and therefore its rarity premium) is important to a profession, but to an economist may be seen as restraint of trade.

THE ECONOMICS OF A PROFESSION

Economists sometimes appear as if they hate professionals. Economists hate specialised expertise. Economists like markets and the free flow of goods and services. They have an inbuilt mistrust of monopolies of any sort. They are likely to mistrust claims to specialised knowledge, which they may see as special pleading, exaggeration of minor differences, a knowledge cartel or as a brazen mechanism of restricting choice and trade, to the disadvantage of consumers. They may characterise a profession as a 'conspiracy against the laity' or as 'vested producer interests'. They will distrust any claims to the nobility of professions and professionals, seeing them as economic arrangements that work to the professional's rather than the public's interest. They may well see professionals as knaves rather than knights.[3]

As John Kay explains in his book *The Truth about Markets*,[4] markets work best when:

- the environment is **competitive**
- the consumer has good knowledge **of available alternatives** and can sensibly make **comparative decisions**
- there is no major **information asymmetry** in favour of either the consumer or the supplier
- the product being bought is a **private good, not a public issue**
- **businesses are free** to define their unique selling points, **'select' their customers, succeed on their merits** and ultimately **go bust if they fail**.

Whether and to what extent the NHS meets any of these criteria, and therefore whether a 'market in healthcare' is a sensible concept, is highly debatable. Although that debate is fascinating, it is best followed in a different forum (see *Putting Patients Last*[5] and 'Should the practice of medicine be a deontological or utilitarian enterprise?'[6]).

Professions contradict most of the principles outlined by Kay. Professions restrict entry to their ranks; they insist on long and rigorous training, and demonstration of skill at the profession; they claim specialised knowledge, which they know well, and which the laity will either not know or not understand well; they claim that the laity trying to do the professional's task will be dangerous and unsafe. The product that professions such as law and medicine provide is both a public good and a private product. It is not provided freely, being subject to much regulation and statutory requirements, which limits the freedom of producers to innovate. The scarcity of professionals reduces competition among them, while guaranteeing them work at a premium price. The collaborative nature of professions and most professionals means that they may be working as much to build relationships with each other as for the public. And they would not see, for example, these two aims as being in conflict – seeing co-operation and collaboration as being good for patients, and the profession.

Most managers (NHS and private) have been trained at least in part in economics and accountancy. They like phrases such as 'allocative efficiency' when describing how resources should be distributed. They can be like Oscar Wilde's cynic, knowing the price of everything and the value of nothing. Whether bringing together the perspectives of managers, who are supposed to know activity and costs, and of clinicians, who are supposed to know the value of the work done into commissioning consortia, is a good strategy remains to be seen. However the alternative of leaving two valid, but unreconciled perspectives in play is unappealing.

There are good reasons why as a consumer or as a manager you may want professionals brought down a peg or two. Professionals are in scarce supply and they cost a lot. If there is a simpler or cheaper alternative then the temptation is to take it. Because of this, there is always a tension between consumers trying to reduce the value of specialised labour and specialised labourers trying to preserve their scarcity and therefore their economic value. The story of the Luddites is especially instructive here. As TW Hanson[7] and EP Thompson[8] narrate, the Luddites were not just bolshie obstructers of progress: they were highly skilled wool processors with a specific skill that took time and trouble to get good at. Their whole skill was devalued to nothing when a new way of processing wool became available, thanks to the engineering genius released at the end of the eighteenth century and to the mill owners who saw the opportunity to do without an expensive part of their labour force. The Luddites were fighting for their livelihoods and their way of life. Now we know from history that they lost this battle, having been totally outflanked by engineering progress. Their story remains instructive to skilled workers in later generations. We would also do well to remember the other guilds of master craftsmen and the many skilled trades and professions that have come and gone over time. From the time frame of history, little is permanent.

For a profession to justify its existence and to refute or mitigate the economist's charges of monopoly and unwarranted restriction of trade, it must show certain characteristics. First, the task it undertakes must be specialised and it must demand a high level of knowledge and skill in its performance. The professional must know much more than the layperson about the task in hand. In short, the profession must establish information asymmetry with its customers. Even with the advent of patient support groups and the availability of much information via Google, there remains an information asymmetry between doctors and their patients. Even the internet printout that a patient arrives with is likely to have been written by another doctor, and may well be a useful refresher for the treating doctor, as well as helpful to the patient.

Second, the profession must define clear and credible standards for entrance to its ranks. This significantly restricts supply, but it increases the quality of the professionals who make up the profession. We know from the research work summarised well by Geoff Colvin in *Talent is Overrated*[9] that the task of becoming good at any skilled task takes a lot of practice over a long period of time. For it to be worth a person putting in the time and effort needed to learn to perform well at their profession, there needs to be some certainty that their efforts will be rewarded. If professionals are not well rewarded they will come to question whether their hard work makes any economic sense and they may well seek to move elsewhere. As my friend Adrian Kenny summarises, any job is an unstable balance of satisfaction, salary and support and although professionals do well on satisfaction and salary, if their support network is reduced, then the compensations of the professional life may not outweigh its hassles.

Third, there must be significant hazard to customers who try to perform the specialised task without professional help. The quote from Red Adair at the beginning of the chapter is helpful here: 'If you think it's expensive to hire a professional to do the job, wait until you hire an amateur.'

Fourth, to justify their protection from the ordinary rules of the market, professionals must be seen to take extra care to put their customer's needs and safety ahead of their own venial concerns. To a large extent, professionals should be noble and self-sacrificing. As the General Medical Council says in *Good Medical Practice*, 'You must make the care of your patient your first concern.'[10]

Fifth, a professional must always be concerned about his or her standards of practice and the quality of their individual and collective efforts. In the recent King's Fund report[11] regarding the quality of UK general practice, there is a criticism of GPs for their failure to fully own and develop the quality agenda in primary care. We think this criticism is partially justified. Any time a professional seems more concerned about his or her own needs, own terms and conditions, or personal interests than about the standards of the care they provide, then they diminish their standing as a professional. When a professional is reduced to saying, 'I only work here', he or she denies their professionalism. Resisting this temptation in a large and complex organisation such as the NHS takes energy and resilience.

Therefore, a profession is justifiable to the extent that it meets these conditions. For me, as an experienced professional, and for my readers, most of whom will be young professionals, it is important to remember the economic and practical justification for professions and the force of the economists' case against professions.

Finally I hope the economists will forgive me for making very broad-brush generalisations about their views in this chapter. I know that in practice their views are more nuanced and variable than those presented starkly here. As doctors we need to remember that economists, whatever their views on the nature of professions and no matter how well they can prepare themselves via Google, will still consult professionals freely if they believe they need our services. They debate, but they are not daft.

REFERENCES

1 Levenson R, Dewar S, Shepherd S. *Understanding Doctors: harnessing professionalism*. London: Royal College of Physicians and King's Fund; 2008. Available at: http://old.rcplondon.ac.uk/professional-Issues/Documents/Understanding-doctors%28Kings-fund%29-FINAL.pdf (accessed 17 December 2011).

2 Bullock A, Trombley S, Lawrie A. *The New Fontana Dictionary of Modern Thought*. 3rd ed./edited by Alan Bullock & Stephen Trombley/assistant editor: Alf Lawrie. London: HarperCollins; 1999.

3 Le Grand J. Knights, knaves or pawns? Human behaviour and social policy. *J Soc Policy*. 1997; **26**(2): 149–69.

4 Kay J. *The Truth about Markets: why some nations are rich but most remain poor*. London: Penguin; 2005.

5 Davies P, Gubb J. *Putting Patients Last*. London: Civitas: Institute for the Study of Civil Society; 2009. Available at: www.civitas.org.uk/pdf/PuttingPatientsLast02July09.pdf (accessed 17 December 2011).

6 Garbutt G, Davies P. Should the practice of medicine be a deontological or utilitarian enterprise? *J Med Ethics*. 2011; **37**(5): 267–70.

7 Hanson TW. *The Story of Old Halifax*. Halifax: F. King & Sons Ltd; 1920.

8 Thompson EP. *The Making of the English Working Class*. London: Penguin; 1963.

9 Colvin G. *Talent is Overrated*. London: Nicholas Brearley Publishing; 2008.

10 GMC. Good Medical Practice. 2009. Available at: www.gmc-uk.org/static/documents/content/GMP_0910.pdf (accessed 11 March 2012).

11 King's Fund. *Improving the Quality of Care in General Practice: report of an independent inquiry commissioned by The King's Fund*. London: The King's Fund; 2011. Available at: www.kingsfund.org.uk/publications/gp_inquiry_report.html (accessed 17 December 2011).

Chapter 3

The primary care landscape

Peter Davies and Lindsay Moran

I would have him learn a little history.
—Oliver Cromwell, to his son's university tutor

What has been will be again, what has been done will be done again;
there is nothing new under the sun.
—Ecclesiastes

Doctors will have more lives to answer for in the next world than
even we generals.
—Napoleon Bonaparte

What is the history of UK general practice? How did we get to where we are? And where are we going in UK general practice?

General practice in the UK has an inspiring history, with many prominent persons shaping its course. Reading this history, one can feel proud to be part of this profession and proud now that general practice in the UK is regarded as one of the world's best. We hope to provide readers with a sense of how general practice has developed, how this explains some of its current features and culture, and to provide some pointers as to how it might develop in the future.

We hope that you as new GPs will play a major part in leading this future, and will make it even better than we foresee.

One of the bad habits of textbooks is just how well they equip their readers to fight the last war but not any future wars. It is difficult for any of us to remember what once we did not know and we tend to take our current knowledge for granted. We are also prone to what is called 'the condescension of posterity'. If you find yourselves tempted to this, remember that the dark ages did not end with the invention of the light bulb, and the Victorians did not live in black and white. The people in the Middle Ages thought of themselves as modern and advanced and did not think they lived in the 'middle' of anything: the term 'Middle Ages' was applied only retrospectively.

We like to imagine that we are clever and young and modern . . . as every generation that has ever lived has also liked to think of themselves. If history teaches us anything, it is to be humble and realise that the same basic problems return in each age, and that we may be just as daft in tackling them as those we look back to.

Veniality, partiality, inability to look forward and to see our own and our patients' best interests will all come into it. The ability to see where everyone else has faultlessly never missed an opportunity to miss an opportunity is great. The reflection that we may be just as good at this as people in the past have been is altogether a much rarer ability.

Remember that many people teach others that which they most need to learn for themselves. Teachers teach a topic because they either consciously or unconsciously know that it is important. In this particular book the authors reserve the right to make bad examples of ourselves every so often. Like politicians who have affairs whilst preaching family values, the authors admit that we may not always perfectly demonstrate all the virtues we describe.

As for the future, we are going to make some predictions about it, but we predict they will be among the first things in this book to become dated.

Here is a very brief sketch of the development of UK general practice, sufficient for current purposes, but we hope accurate enough for it to avoid disappearing into the mists of Tannochbrae, where Dr Finlay is apparently still practising, and Janet is still serving the tea. (For those new to Dr Finlay, he was the fictional hero from the TV series *Dr Finlay's Casebook* (1962–71), based on the novel *Country Doctor* by AJ Cronin. Dr Finlay worked in the Scottish town of Tannochbrae during the 1920s and knew all his patients well, from cradle to grave, and thus was his fame.)

GENERAL PRACTICE . . . THE EVOLUTION
The dark ages
Medicine in these times was very different from how we know it today. It was a private transaction between you and your customer. The profession and the market were unregulated, and the patients operated on a basis of *caveat emptor* – 'let the buyer beware!' Medicine was a good or product to be traded in the market place. It was transactional, and doctors had to compete for customers

with many others: quacks, folk healers, herbalists and many more. (Indeed, this was how the barber surgeons established their trade, by cutting more than just their clients' hair!) There was no superstructure, little specialisation, and medical transactions were private, commercial transactions, and so confidentiality was inbuilt – to the patient and the family. Illness was largely a private tragedy and, except in the cases of epidemics, there was no one else who needed to know about it. The cause of illness often had a superstitious or religious basis and so, therefore, did the treatments (e.g. bloodletting to release the 'bad humours').

For the rich patients with adequate finance, they had a free choice of service, but it may not have been very effective, even if expensive. Care for the poor was limited, although some charitable medical care was provided by the churches and monasteries.

In some ways this practice had its benefits – there were no government targets or Quality and Outcomes Framework to contend with, but, equally, evidence-based medicine was barely considered, although medical ethics and standards were beginning to become important.

Gradually there came to be some regulation and standard setting. The colleges of physicians and surgeons were established in 1518 and 1540 respectively, and these colleges started to set specific standards for membership.

Medical knowledge advanced massively over the seventeenth, eighteenth and nineteenth centuries. Gradually more colleges and universities were founded, and by the mid-nineteenth century it became necessary to recognise medicine as a specific profession with specific entry requirements in the Medical Act of 1858. This act recognised 'duly qualified medical practitioners' and distinguished them sharply from lay or untrained other healers. It laid specific duties and obligations on doctors, but it also gave them the specific legal definition unique to the profession.

There was a growing awareness during the nineteenth century that medicine was a part of society, and that it could not just focus on treating those who presented to its practitioners for care. In 1842, Edwin Chadwick's report on the condition of the poor in Manchester raised the profile of the differences between rich and poor in health outcomes, and of how great a disease burden the lower classes lived with.

The awareness of infection and its risk of contagion meant that the connections between personal and societal conditions had to be made. Perhaps the pinnacle of such work was the realisation stated clearly by German pathologist Rudolf Virchow that 'Medicine is a social science, and politics is nothing else but medicine on a large scale.' Virchow plainly saw the diseases in his patients as a sign of disease within the wider body politic of his society. The classic example of this is the physician John Snow's work in revealing the Broad Street pump as the source of the cholera contagion in the Broad Street area of London in 1854.

The great public health and social reforms of the Victorian age – factory acts, clean water supplies and so on – began to have an impact on health, and awareness that social conditions had a great impact on health began to grow. Medical officers of health became an important bridge between local medical practice and local social policies. Medicine was realised to be as much a social science as about treating disease.

It was around this time when general practice first established itself as a profession. A number of doctors broke away from the hospital consultant fraternities and went to treat patients in the community. Towards the end of the nineteenth century the UK had a pattern of GPs, surgeons and physicians. It also had care provision in three main categories: (1) at home, (2) in the hospital or (3) in the workhouse.

The late 1800s and early 1900s

People realised that they needed protection from illness and treatment for it. They realised illness was sporadic, somewhat unpredictable, devastating for finances and expensive to treat. Very few people (then and now) had the finances set aside to provide for treatment of illness as it occurred. The Victorians developed an insurance system that involved paying a subscription in return for benefits when sick. This was the origin of worker health associations, the factory-based 'panel' doctors and, therefore, the GP's list-based care of patients. The role of GPs was given a boost by their recognition in David Lloyd George's National Insurance Act of 1911. Working men could now register on a GP's 'panel' and this GP would receive an annual capitation fee to care for them – at least this improved health for those at work in the nation.

The downside of this was the role of the doctor not just in treating the patient but also in providing reports for government benefits. The sick note (Med3 and its new replacement, the fit note) all stem from this time. The ability of the doctor to issue sick notes and recommendations for other benefits has over time spawned many spin-offs; some useful extra work for GPs and some burdensome. The GANFYD (Get A Note From Your Doctor) phenomenon is a direct offshoot of this work, and a current pest in our surgeries driving people to see us for reasons other than medical care. It has led to the phenomenon of an illness not as something to recover from but as a means to financial and other benefits. History is moving full circle, and the government is currently (November 2011) looking to remove the burden of providing long-term sickness certification from GPs, and this relief will be welcome to many GPs.

Generally GPs in this time worked single-handed and to top up capitation fees, their services were mainly charged for.

Alongside the social changes, medical knowledge was growing, and being concentrated in hospitals. 'Disease palaces' was their affectionate term, but hospitals were the place where medical knowledge was growing the fastest. The development of anaesthetics allowed surgeons to operate further and more deeply; the pathologists got their hands on ever more material from operations and post-mortems; generalist physicians were becoming more specialised or being displaced by specialists. Certain illnesses had such stigma that the doctors who care for such patients had to work in specialised isolated units, hence how specialised hospitals such as The National Hospital for Diseases of the Nervous System including Paralysis and Epilepsy came to be needed.

The GP was always busy with a large list of patients to see, and he had little time for learning the new developments that were being made in the teaching hospitals. The literature of medicine was hospital dominated and written, and primary care had little or no narrative or justification of its own. It was just busy. The characters are vividly summarised in George Bernard Shaw's play *The Doctor's Dilemma*, with the contrasts among Sir Ralph Bloomfield Bonington (surgeon), Sir Colenso Ridgeon (physician) and Dr Blenkinsop (GP) being very sharply drawn.

Over time the division between in-hospital and out-of-hospital care became sharper, in administrative and clinical knowledge and capability terms. The hospital was seen as the centre of medical knowledge and practice, and primary care became partially detached from this. Sir Clifford Allbutt, a hospital physician, summarised primary care as the 'perfunctory work . . . of perfunctory men'.

However, the hospital systems were overwhelmed with demand and they started insisting on a referral process. Hospital doctors would only see patients at their emergency rooms if they had a letter of recommendation from the primary care physician. Thus 'gatekeeping' began and such was the origin of the referral system in UK medicine – as a means of demand management, rather than as a planned piece of care system planning. This feature of ad hoc solutions being turned into long-term systems without planning or thought for the overall picture is a recurring theme of UK health services provision.

The 1940s

In 1948, in the aftermath of the war years, the NHS was born. It was born from the ideal that all should be able to receive healthcare, regardless of wealth. It was, and still is, a tremendous expression of shared social values and an acceptance of a need by all of society, from richest to poorest, to contribute to a pooled risk fund to pay for the provision of medical and other healthcare. Universal coverage is a great achievement that we should value very highly. With free care available to all, GPs could concentrate their care from cradle to grave. GPs had remained partially outside the NHS in 1948, preferring to remain as small businessmen rather than becoming salaried primary care doctors, and this model continues to this day. The pros and cons of this are still being reviewed. (For the current generation of doctors this will certainly be reviewed again. At some stage in the next 10–20 years will most UK GPs move from being partners to being salaried employees?)

General practice was still very much a 'cottage industry' at the time of the formation of the NHS. It had issues of variability, availability and coverage but otherwise it was in a reasonable state. However, the introduction of free healthcare for all impacted greatly upon the burden of workload for GPs, who did not have the physical, administrative or financial resources to cope. Workload was large. Standards dropped. Morale fell. General practice was at a crisis point.

The workings of the inverse care law was readily observable, although the phenomenon was not named until Tudor-Hart defined it in his 1971 *Lancet* paper:

> The availability of good medical care tends to vary inversely with the need for it in the population served. This inverse care law operates more completely where medical care is most exposed to market forces, and less so where such exposure is reduced.[1]

The 1950s

The Collings report of 1950[2] exposed the problems of much UK general practice; indeed, there were questions as to whether it was worth keeping the specialty at all. The report exposed poor medicine being practised in poor surroundings by undertrained doctors. It showed problems with the organisation of services, and flaws in the processes of care. It showed a demoralised group of doctors with little in the way of incentives for improvement or optimism. It was a damning and accurate report.

Under all this strain, it was proposed by a group of leading GPs that a College for General Practitioners be formed to influence good medical standards of practice, education and research (400 years after the medical and surgical colleges were formed – this seemed long overdue!). Thus a 'steering committee' formed and worked to gain college status – their aim, to provide leadership and better standards in general practice. Sir Henry Willink, the former minister of health (1943–45), Master of Magdalene College, Cambridge, chaired the meetings.

Following only eight meetings, the College of General Practitioners was founded as a charitable organisation in November 1952 with legal constitution, despite opposition from colleges based on secondary care. Its role was to provide an 'academic headquarters for general practice and to raise the standards and status of general practice'. It was to provide intellectual and educational leadership to the profession, and lay down far-reaching frameworks around what good general practice is and what GPs should be working towards. An article published in the *Practitioner* at this time said it is 'an outstanding event in the history of British medicine'. So, despite an initial lukewarm reception, the start of the college was heralded as a great triumph for general practice, with much written support sent in from many practising GPs, delighted with the advent of the honourable college ideals.

The college defined membership criteria for entry and within 6 weeks it had over 1600 members. Gradually various committees were formed – undergraduate, postgraduate and research. Regional faculties were created to give local responsibility to advance college aims. The reports and publications from this time make it clear that the college was an influential academic body.

The 1960s and 1970s

These were good times for the college. The coat of arms was patented in 1961.

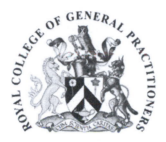

The symbols are:

- the gavel entwined with the serpent (representing the staff of Asclepius, the Greek god of healing)
- the shield (black/white) representing day and night, alluding to the 24-hour commitment of GPs to their patients
- the owl, symbolising enlightenment, and the lamp, symbolising wide-ranging knowledge
- the white poppy, symbolising the relief of pain, and the blue gentian, representing palliative care.

In 1962 the college purchased the headquarters in Princes Gate, London, for £175 000 (selling it in 2010 for rather more).

In 1965 the college held the first MRCGP examination for membership to its ranks. The higher-class membership of fellowship was first awarded in 1967 to award members who had contributed greatly to general practice.

No discipline that wants to be taken seriously can neglect its own epistemology – its own specific knowledge, and its own way of knowing about the world. Until 1972 there was no specific training for general practice; it was assumed that a medical degree based on hospital-acquired knowledge was sufficient for becoming a GP. In 1972 this notion was challenged, and the need for specific vocational training for general practice became established. The basic structure of 2 years in hospital posts and 1 year in a training practice became established. Parliament passed legislation approving compulsory vocational training for all GPs, which had been successfully campaigned for through the Todd report from 1968.[3]

The Royal College of General Practitioners was born in 1972 when the college was presented its royal charter with HRH The Prince Philip, Duke of Edinburgh, appointed as Honorary Fellow and president of the college. He has since relinquished the role to be the college's patron.

In this same year the college also published a book titled *The Future General Practitioner*. When you read this you will see the first description of ideas that can now be taken for granted; ideas around future GPs looking at bio-psychosocial consultations, patient centeredness, proper training and end point assessment, revalidation at intervals are all anticipated in this book. A lot of the ideas about which you will probably think, 'Oh, that's what all GPs think' were predicted in this book, although it has taken 40 years for those ideas to be worked into our systems.

The 1980s, 1990s and 2000s

Like all institutions the college was restructured a few times and more divisions established, with positive aims; services to members and faculties, clinical and research and education with an examination board were established.

Methods of teaching and training for prospective GPs evolved. For training it had initially been thought that it was enough to simply turn up for the jobs and be noted as having attended. In time the need for an explicit end point assessment became obvious, and after much struggle and debate this was introduced as a summative assessment in 1994. The summative assessment ran in parallel with the MRCGP exam, which, sadly, was not merged with summative assessment. This has led to the phenomenon of there being many current, and often senior, GPs who have passed their summative assessment but have not bothered with MRCGP; sadly, this leaves a pool of talented GPs outside the college and its activities.

THE MEMBERSHIP OF THE ROYAL COLLEGE OF GENERAL PRACTITIONERS EXAMINATION AND BEYOND

Eventually the college and the General Practitioners Committee got GP registrars to reach a common end point of training recognised by college membership – hence nMRCGP from 2008 onwards with the delightful ePortfolio, the Applied Knowledge Test and the much-feared Clinical Skills Assessment. Despite the embarrassment, video consultations were to stay as well, the benefits of recording one's own consultations being well recognised.

The college tends to provide a lot of influence around our feelings about what should happen in general practice, and the British Medical Association's General Practitioners Committee tries to capture this in contracts some years later. For example, the contractual support and encouragement for moving towards group practices in the 1966 GP contract came out of the intellectual view that single-handed practice was not the best way to do general practice. More recently, although ideas about 'opportunistic health promotion' had been around for many years (at least since 1975), it was only with the advent of the Quality and Outcomes Framework in the new General Medical Services contract in 2004 that it became contractually important to do it.

The RCGP is now the largest of the medical royal colleges, with a membership of over 42 000. With its motto being *Cum Scientia Caritas*, 'Knowledge with compassion', it responds to political ideas, shouting them down or occasionally praising them; it has branched out into international waters, holds conferences for its members, publishes journals, has entrance exams to guarantee standards and leads on primary care research. Prior to the advent of the college in 1952, doubts to the survival of general practice as a profession were commonly heard. In 2009 a survey across 10 000 primary care doctors carried out by US think tank the Commonwealth Fund concluded that British primary care is the best in the world. We are cost-effective for the nation, delivering an excellent service for our patients and avoiding the need for expensive secondary care involvement. Also, nations with an effective primary care system have lower morbidity and mortality rates – an overall great outcome from the apprehensive beginnings.

THE PITFALLS OF THE NATIONAL HEALTH SERVICE

From the strengths of the college's early days to the present, we could not consider this in context without considering that the NHS and general practice has not been without its pitfalls as well. As much as we all strive to work to our best in our field, the waters that we are in are rather murky.

We have seen a supposedly national service become a fixed-cost envelope within which distribution of resources has been uneven and skewed, leading to the current state where we have vastly different levels of services delivered and standards achieved across the UK. The NHS may be national, but as experienced by patients it is variable, parochial and often driven by fissures between departments and services. The silos of secondary care, teaching hospitals, social services and primary care have all been deepened by successive NHS changes. I remember being at a local medical committee meeting one time and at the end of the negotiation the hospital's medical director said, 'I accept your points but surely we are all in this for the same thing, aren't we?' Sadly, the answer to his question was 'No', because of the rules of finance and contract of each of the silos we were arguing from.

The NHS has been massively centralised. This should lead to consistency and fair distribution of resources but, sadly, the opposite has been the case. The NHS has been unable to respond quickly to change, and to move providers of care to where they are needed. I suppose it puts it into perspective when you consider that the NHS is the world's fourth-largest employer (beaten only by the Chinese Army, the Indian Railway and Wal-Mart). The NHS has rarely had either the intelligence to make such decisions or the ability to act on such information even if it were available. The distribution of teaching hospitals within London is a stark example of this failing. The inverse care law is a stark consequence of this fact.

In fact, the NHS has largely removed the local voice from healthcare, with even regional (strategic) and local health authorities (primary care trusts) being run largely as outposts of the centre, rather than as advocates for localities. The NHS has long had a culture of central credit and local blame and this has sapped the initiative of local management in most of the NHS for many years. And there is a local democratic deficit (pre-1948 the councils and other local bodies were directly concerned about their local hospitals, as they ran them. After 1948 the local voice in healthcare was muted, being replaced by trusted appointees of the centre). Decisions about provision of services that matter intensely locally are often taken miles away at the Department of Health in London. The NHS is in sharp contrast to the rest of Europe, where the provision of services is much more locally focused. Aneurin Bevan's memorable phrase about the dropped bedpan echoing down the corridors of Whitehall would be greeted with incredulity in most of Europe. There the dropped bedpan would echo no further than the end of the ward, and the sister or the local managers would have absolute authority to sort it out.

There is a fear of being overwhelmed by demand that is a recurring theme in UK medicine. Once we are aware of unmet needs and the finite nature of medical systems, at our personal level and at the wider corporate level, then we fear that finding unmet needs may lead to so much demand on the system that it will not be able to cope, having insufficient money, people or equipment to provide the treatment necessary. This has been the 'sky falling moment' for many secretaries of state for health as the waiting lists get too long to be bearable. Our responses to this fear are rarely fully rational, either individually or collectively, and we rarely plan services from area-wide knowledge of the extent of the problem and the extent of the resource. This leads to partially informed and often short-sighted solutions that are temporary fixes that often last rather longer than is sensible. You will be able to spot many of these in the NHS in both primary and secondary care, and part of your work as new GPs will be to recognise that these need not continue into the future.

The 'way it is around here' may well be an accident, not a well-designed function. In terms of workforce planning, these mismatches between need and resource often lead to new training opportunities that, when the training is complete, open up onto a problem now past. Think of upper gastrointestinal surgeons and peptic ulcer operations after the significance of *Helicobacter pylori* became apparent.

We see from this consideration the origin of one of the recurring debates around general practice. This is about the extent to which general practice should be about the individual patient as an end in themselves, and the extent to which it should be the front line of public health measures to make the wider society better and safer. Behind this come the echoes of the debates about the one vs. the many, the duties and rights of individuals vs. their responsibilities and duties to society, confidentiality vs. public disclosure, the Rose paradox (*see* Chapter 19) and many more. The balance of these twin tracks – the individual and their host society – shift over time, and they will shift again, but the two themes will likely remain waxing and waning against each other. Both approaches are necessary, but the balance between them is never settled. How you relate to these themes will determine how you are as a doctor, how you will practise, and what kind of attitude you will take when the issues are debated.

General practices themselves are ripe for change. The current system of small, scattered partnerships may not be the best configuration for providing primary care, for either patients or doctors. The lack of coordination among the parts of primary care (e.g. GP surgery, podiatrists, the ambulance service) is unhelpful. Why is the local A&E department not considered part of primary care and integrated with it? Why was NHS Direct not integrated with anything?

GP partnerships may need to reappraise their structure and function, and consider moving towards becoming 'medical services provider organisations' and thinking of themselves as businesses that provide high standards of service to meet specified needs. 'General practice' may not be a specific enough description of what we can do in the future. Expect to see business development managers as a key part of your practice in the future, and expect to be working closely with them to define exactly what services you provide well and to whom. The old 'John Wayne' contract of 'A GP's gotta do what a GP does' has largely gone, and we will need to be much clearer in future about what we offer and about who is buying our service. Expect to regard processes of bidding and tendering as routine business in the future (some practices already do).

There has long been a false equivalence drawn between 'NHS spending' and 'health achieved for population'. This leads to a Dutch auction in which politicians feel that they have to pledge to spend more on 'Health' without distinguishing between what the NHS does (remedial healthcare) and what the desired outcome is – namely, a more healthy population. The contribution of the NHS to health is at best partial. To have allowed our society's necessary political discourse and debate on what health is and how to achieve it for individuals and as a society to be reduced to who can pay for a few more or a few less operations is an intellectual impoverishment that doctors, patients and politicians should all be ashamed of.

The NHS has never really understood performance issues. The NHS has never really understood itself as a system that operates on inputs to produce results. Instead, the NHS has understood itself as a series of tasks, often best broken down into parts and dealt with separately. This was carried severely to absurdity by the last government, with its regime of 'targets and terror' and, for example, 4-hour waits being achieved in A&E departments while ambulances were stacked up outside waiting to unload patients. Expect performance specification and measurement to become routine. Add the Donabedian triad of 'structure, process and outcome' to your vocabulary, alongside 'ideas, concerns and expectations'.

As far as we can tell (either then or now, using UK or international viewpoints), raising the money to pay for healthcare by taxation is as fair a way of paying for healthcare costs as any. (The alternatives are direct payments by patients, mixed revenue raising by means of national taxes, local taxes, taxes on employers, user charges or insurance systems. None of these have any great advantage over any other – however you decide to pay for it, healthcare is expensive, and the cost has to be paid somewhere by someone.)

Effectively, the UK NHS is currently a £1600 per person per year pooled risk, state-held healthcare insurance fund.

The UK NHS is described as being triple nationalised: it has one funding stream (taxation), one channel of distribution (via the Department of Health and its regional offshoots) and one system of provision (via NHS doctors, nurses and other suppliers). This system has certain strengths in that for many years it kept administration costs down, kept most doctors away from commerce, kept overall costs down and meant that each part of the system was part of a greater whole. However, there are many weaknesses of the system that were inbuilt in 1948 and which have become magnified over time. Successive secretaries of state have wrestled mightily with these weaknesses over the last 60 years, and has finally (March 2012) just gone through parliament.

Seasoned NHS watchers will now be going 'until the next one'. If NHS history teaches you anything it is that change is constant, and that change is not the same as progress. As a young GP you may well be swept up in the enthusiasm for the next great change. The pattern seems to be, for both doctors and managers, that you enjoy the first one you experience, see some good points in the second, spot the bad points in the third, and yearn for retirement by the fourth. As an example of the personal impact this can have for NHS workers, a Yorkshire public health director has had to reapply for his job six times in the last 14 years. There's never been any doubt that the job was his, but he has been distracted with curricula vitae and interviews when he need not have been. He's borne the process with private frustration and public fortitude. Many others have had similar experiences.

Sadly, the nationalisation of the health service left unchallenged some features of the medical landscape that really should have been uprooted at the inception of the service. There has rarely been any systematic thought about 'What would a good service to patients look like? Followed by 'And so what resources need to go where to achieve this?' Instead we have seen fire-fighting and infighting among the parts of the service, which have collectively put more effort into infighting and protecting their silos than into forging common purpose. The whole has achieved far less than it could and should have done throughout its history. Too many people have been employed to work within frames of reference from which the only sensible strategy for them was to get as much of the NHS pie as they could for their department, and pay no heed to the overall good of the system. Those doctors and managers who should have been holding the ring against such partisanship have been underpowered and under-supported by the centre. The new commissioning bodies appearing since 2011 are the latest attempt to produce a powerful-enough NHS commissioning function to counterbalance the problem of supplier-dictated activity with accurate specification of what a patient-focused service would actually look like.

Anyway, the UK's NHS is as it is, and as new GPs you will have to find some way of making sense of what is going on around you. There are many frames of reference ready for major rewriting if you are brave enough.

AND THE FUTURE?

The current UK NHS primary and secondary care landscapes are shifting significantly. With this come both the threats and opportunities open to existing and new GPs. Some of you will like the changes and some of you will not. Either way, you will not avoid them. GPs see patients for 9 out of 10 of their contacts with all doctors, and thus the personal, social and political importance of our professional work is huge, and probably about to increase. However the NHS evolves, we know that strong primary care will make the whole system work better, and perhaps it is now time for the generalist perspective to be stated more strongly than it has been previously.

You as a young GP will play a part in how the history unfolds.

REFERENCES

1 Hart JT. The inverse care law. *Lancet*. 1971 Feb 27; **1**(7696): 405–12.
2 Collings JS. General practice in England today: a reconnaissance. *Lancet* 1950; **i**: 555–85.

3 Townsend E. Royal Commission on Medical Education 1965–68 report. *J R Coll Gen Pract.* 1968 September; **16**(3): 245–7.

FURTHER READING

In this chapter we have given a very brief sketch of the development of the primary care system in the UK. The books listed in this section will give you a far fuller picture of our profession and our own specialty and how they have emerged and developed. The King's Fund, Health Foundation and RCGP references define the current challenges we face, and lay down the clinical and managerial challenge facing us that will keep us busy in the next 10 years.

- Cronin AJ. *The Citadel.* Boston: Little, Brown and Co; 1937. A powerful novel that captures an early phase of modern general practice. Superbly describes the development of a young doctor as he comes to terms with his profession and its work. Sadly, the phenomenon of 'assistant with (a rather distant) view of partnership' seems to be reappearing in modern UK general practice.
- Health Foundation, Royal College of General Practitioners. *Guiding Patients through Complexity: modern medical generalism.* London; 2011. Available at: www.health. org.uk/public/cms/75/76/4299/2763/COMMISSION%20REPORT%20ON%20 MEDICAL%20GENERALISM%20OCTOBER%202011.pdf?realName=xbuUe5. pdf (accessed 17 December 2011). A superb examination of the concept of generalism and its strengths and weaknesses.
- King's Fund. *Improving the Quality of Care in General Practice: report of an independent inquiry commissioned by The King's Fund.* London: The King's Fund; 2011. Available at: www.kingsfund.org.uk/publications/gp_inquiry_report.html (accessed 17 December 2011). The current challenge to our profession; nicely expressed, but with some significant nudges about things we as GPs need to improve.
- Klein R. *The New Politics of the NHS: from creation to reinvention.* 6th ed. Oxford: Radcliffe Publishing; 2010. A classic book, regularly updated. Your understanding of how the NHS works is increased significantly if you read this book.
- Lawrence C. *Medicine in the Making of Modern Britain 1700–1920.* Historical Connections Series. London: Routledge; 1994. Short and good at linking the past to the present.
- Misselbrook D. *Thinking about Patients.* Newbury: Petroc Press; 2001. An insightful examination of what patients want and need at many different levels and perspectives; a wise, encouraging, thought-provoking and tolerant book.
- Porter R. *Greatest Benefit to Mankind: a medical history of humanity from antiquity to the present.* London: HarperCollins; 1997. An excellent book. All of human death and dying and what doctors have tried to do about it is here – a wide and generous perspective.
- Royal College of General Practitioners. *The Future General Practitioner.* London:

RCGP; 1972. Who sets the frame sets the game, and this book has been setting the frames of reference around our profession for the last 40 years.

- Seddon N. *Quite Like Heaven: options for the NHS in a consumer age*. London: Civitas: Institute for the Study of Civil Society; 2007.
- Shaw GB. *The Doctor's Dilemma*. New York: Penguin; 1902. An interesting view of medicine. The preface is an excellent review of medicine and its travails; the play is fun, and has some well-drawn medical archetypes.
- Sheard S, Donaldson L. *The Nation's Doctor: the role of the chief medical officer 1855–1998*. Oxford: Radcliffe Publishing; 2006. Surprisingly readable, and a great introduction to key medical leaders over time.
- Tudor-Hart JT. *A New Kind of Doctor: the general practitioner's part in the health of the community*. London: Merlin Press; 1988. A superb vision of what general practice could and maybe should be like. Good understanding about how UK general practice came to be how it is.
- Webster C. *The National Health Service: a political history*. Oxford: Oxford University Press; 2002. Witty and acerbic.

Chapter **4**

The work of general practice

Peter Davies, with input from Lindsay Moran

WHAT IS THE WORK OF GENERAL PRACTICE?

The extent of the profession: what should the work of a GP be?

When you think of general practice, what do you think GPs are doing? Almost immediately most of you will answer that GPs are busy seeing patients. For most GPs this is exactly what they are doing, and exactly what they should be doing. However, many GPs also fill other roles that are valid and useful. For new GPs it is worth being aware of these options, enlarging your perspective on what the role of the GP is and realising just how many roles are open to GPs. You may want to incorporate one or many of these other roles into your portfolio in the future. Even if you do not take any of them on, it is at least worth realising these roles exist, knowing what purpose they serve, and appreciating your colleagues who have moved into them.

Combining too many of these roles at once is problematic, both individually and for partnership dynamics. However there is a strong case for seeing the work of general practice as being about far more than just surgeries full of patients. In future I think we will see general practice conceived and described in a wider way than it currently is, both by outsiders (our patients and our commissioners) and by us ourselves. Quite how practices will adapt to this is currently uncertain, although the usual rule is that British GPs eventually adapt to anything, albeit with loud mutters along the way.

GP consultations

Most GPs are busy each day seeing many patients who 'either are or believe themselves to be ill'. They do this in GP surgeries as part of small business organisations (GP partnerships) or via the increasing number of medical service companies that are now running GP surgeries.

However you look at it, GPs exist to serve patients and they do this by meeting patients in the consulting room and making some sense of the patient's symptoms, diagnosis and treatment. Even though we think of GP consultations as occurring in a surgery, many now take place in other venues such as walk-in centres, out-of-hours services and sometimes the patient's home. In the United States some GPs take it a step further and visit their patients in hospital to do their own ward rounds. So too do some rural GPs in remote areas with cottage hospitals in the UK. And we may see an intermediate care tier opening up in the UK NHS that will need significant planned primary care input, and more than just sporadic GP visits.

Running a practice

Practices do not run themselves. They run well because someone makes this happen. To bring in income, surgeries need to have a specialised development and leadership role within the practice that allows one of the doctors to take time out from clinical work to make sure this happens. You will need to learn some element of business skills. There is a duty on all of us to support efforts to improve the quality of our services. There is a lot of work here, and if it is not specifically planned into the working week it will not happen. As is so often true, 'failing to plan is planning to fail'.

GP with a special interest

GP with a special interest (GPwSI) is an option for some GPs. It provides an outlet for additional medical skills or it allows you to learn more about an area of medicine. Some GPs loathe the concept of GPwSI on the grounds that we are generalists through and through, and any hint of specialisation is unwelcome. In other cases GPs have got themselves a more varied life, combining routine surgeries with additional work such as echocardiography, endoscopy, dermatology, minor surgery and so on. Often these extra roles add interest to the GP's life and bring extra ideas into the practice. They can increase the range and depth of relationships these GPs have. In the new world of commissioning, some of these activities could become useful commissioned enhanced services from the practice, and therefore bring extra income into the practice.

There are many options for GPwSI work, and different areas have used them in different ways. For example, in Bradford these roles were strongly encouraged and many GPs developed into them, but in nearby Calderdale these roles have hardly been used at all.

Academic options

Academic options basically fall into two broad camps: teaching and researching.

The main teaching roles are undergraduate teaching and postgraduate GP training. There is a lot of work to be done under both these headings. Different doctors and different practices differ in the extent to which they want to be involved in these options. Many doctors come to love teaching and training and it becomes a major part of who they are as a doctor. If you are keen at exploring teaching roles, speak with your local VTS or academic unit at the local medical school.

The main research roles are within university departments, but the split between 'service' and 'research' is too big at present and many university departments are looking to bring local GPs and their practices into their work. Schemes such as Research Ready allow practices the option of participating in research with university colleagues.

For those who want to lead research then the first step is to move in such a way as to be able to get a research degree completed. Speak to local university departments and professors about exact requirements. College faculties are often a good place to meet people with these interests.

Medical politics

The local medical committee (LMC), the British Medical Association and the RCGP all have key roles in how medical practice is run and managed in the UK. They operate at local and national levels and at the very least it is worth knowing what these bodies do. If you find the work fascinating then you can make a major contribution to your local colleagues by working with these bodies and you will personally gain the understanding of the background operations to the general practice world and how it coexists with current political thinking.

Commissioning

Commissioning is the new big thing for GPs. It looks like it is going to be a major feature of the NHS landscape for many years to come. It is taking a lot of clinical input to run. For example, in Calderdale there are 130 GPs on the performers list and 10 of these are on the commissioning consortium. The hours they are contracted for are equivalent to about an extra three full-time GPs. This is a major new role that has come the way of the GP, and it is a fascinating opportunity for leadership and additional work within primary care. Furthermore, often within each practice now a practice lead for commissioning is appointed and this will take 27 half-day sessions of doctor time each week – equivalent to another three full-time GPs. Similar figures are coming out in other areas across the country. Commissioning is a major demand on the profession locally and nationally, and it is taking experienced GPs into new roles. It is also creating demand for locum doctors as backfill.

Quality control: appraisal and revalidation, medical directors and responsible officers

There is now a more explicit recognition that the quality of medical care needs to be assessed, measured and improved. Over the last 10 years we have seen the emergence of the medical appraisal system, the move to revalidation, and new roles in local primary care such as appraisers, appraisal leads and medical directors. Once revalidation is launched, responsible (for performance) officers will emerge. This work is crucial to improving the quality and consistency of primary care, and to trying to reduce unwarranted variations between doctors and practices. This work is likely to expand over time and create more vacancies for GPs. It is interesting and important work.

Specific niche areas: substance misuse, prison work, homelessness, special projects

There have always been areas or groups of patients who get a poor deal from established services. For example, homeless people struggle to register with a GP, as they have no address. In many urban areas the primary care trust has set up specific homeless projects.

People in prisons have many health needs, both physical and mental, and the recent improvements in prison healthcare systems are to be welcomed.

Substance misuse services have expanded significantly over the last 10 years or so and they have helped enormously in dealing with the problem of addiction. Most of the doctors working in this field are GPs who have moved into the area, not psychiatrists. These doctors have helped their regular colleagues by neutralising the problem of addiction. When I started in practice in the 1990s, requests for '100 of those nice DF118 tablets' were commonplace (maybe one request per week); these days I very rarely get addicts trying such requests on (once a year or less now).

Some areas have GPs who specialise in managing patients in residential and nursing homes.

All of these niche areas may become an opportunity for a new GP. Your best way of discovering more about these areas is to speak to the doctors already working in them.

Sideways moves into occupational health, public health or health screening

GP training is often a good starting point for other specialties. For example, many GPs move (after extra training) into public health work. Some move into occupational health work, some move into adult or child psychiatry, and others move into work such as health screening. All of these roles can be interesting to some GPs – it is all useful medicine.

Forces medical services

Soldiers may be fit and healthy, but they need a good medical service to keep them that way. Military medicine can range from routine to the excitement and risk of battlefield medicine. Soldiers have specific needs, and there is a knack to doing military medicine well. If it appeals to you it could become a good career for you.

Medical journalism

Many doctors write well. There are papers for the public and there are trade magazines such as *GP* and *Pulse* that need good copy from good writers. If you can write well then there are opportunities to contribute here. These days there are opportunities with local and national papers and via many websites. If you read this kind of material and think you could contribute to it, then get writing, get commissioned and see how you do. Most medical journalists combine their writing with part-time practice – it's difficult to keep writing about a job you no longer do. At least medicine always has some interesting events and people to generate good copy from.

Medical defence organisations, other medico-legal work, expert witness

There is much work these days in the medico-legal field. Most of us contact our medical defence organisations for advice periodically. The doctors who answer our calls and calm our fears are experienced doctors acting as medico-legal advisers. They are often drawn from a general practice background.

There is much other medico-legal work too. Negligence may be bad for the doctor being complained about, but it creates work for other doctors in commenting on the case and clarifying the issues involved. Becoming an expert witness, whether for defence or the prosecution, can be a rewarding niche in general practice.

The compensation culture is creating demand for independent medical examiners to assess injuries and their severity. Some GPs have made a niche for themselves doing this work.

The General Medical Council needs case examiners to assess complaints, panellists for fitness to practise hearings, and specialty advisors to the panels.

Advisory roles and capacity assessments

Many organisations such as government bodies, the Department of Health, the National Institute for Health and Clinical Excellence, Connecting for Health and so on need decent medical advice to help them to develop decent policy. There is work here for GPs (among others); some of it is well paid and some not.

Other work includes capacity assessments for benefits (e.g. employment and support allowances). The UK benefits system is complex, and a lot of its work involves separating worthy from unworthy claimants for benefits. Which person is severely disabled by their illness? Which one could manage to go back to work? There is a lot of work for doctors to perform the assessments that help make such decisions.

Private GP work

Private GP work can be an enjoyable way of working for some doctors. The option is more open in London than elsewhere. It is hard work, and has some benefits and some problems compared with routine NHS general practice. Expect to work hard, and to have to constantly think about how your service adds value to your clients. Some doctors like thinking in this business-oriented manner.

As you can see from the list of roles outlined in this chapter so far (and I am sure this list is not exhaustive) there are many roles beyond the consulting room and the traditional practice that your GP training opens up to you. These additional roles sometimes become full-time in their own right, and some can be combined with work in the surgery (a portfolio career). Most would prefer GPs with some experience, so as a new GP you may need to do preliminary work rather than apply for the job immediately. Many of these roles need significant extra training to do them well.

The number of roles opening up to GPs is increasing. These roles will either appeal to you or help create vacancies (sessional and permanent) back in the surgeries as mid-career GPs take on additional roles and responsibilities.

With this many options open to us as a specialty the question is not 'is there a job?' but 'are there enough of us to do all the work that needs doing?' Finding work with your GP qualification should be no problem at all.

There are many niches within general practice. At least one of them is likely to suit you. As Flanders and Swann put it in their song 'The Gasman Cometh', 'It all makes work for the working man to do'. These days we need to add 'and woman'.

Taking on roles outside your regular clinical practice can be immensely satisfying. And how do you get to take part in these various roles? Occasionally the role will fall your way by sheer chance, being in the right place, at the right time with the right person. But if that is not the case for you, then you need to be more proactive. Contact your local university and see what opportunities there are for you. Contact your local medical committee or faculty to ask if you can attend as an observer. Usually all these places are delighted to have a keen person attend. The same goes for commissioning roles. If you are interested in GPwSI work, then discuss this with GPwSIs doing the role at present – ask how they got into it. Look into doing a diploma if necessary or doing clinics alongside a hospital consultant. Even simply doing a search for what you want to do on Google can be useful. You may need to contact companies directly for certain roles, i.e. for working as a ship doctor, or for private insurance work. Whatever the case may be, if you have an interest, then look into it and give it a go.

YOUR PORTFOLIO OF ROLES OVER TIME

One of the things British medicine has been bad at in the past is that once it has people trained for a role, it assumes that these people stay in that role forever; for example, 'a GP'. There has been relatively little discussion and thought given to what exactly 'a GP' is, and what it is exactly that he or she should do. There has been little thought given as to how the role should change over time, yet, for example, my 57-year-old male senior partner has different hopes and aspirations from me, and from my younger 36-year-old female partner. We are all covered by the term 'GP', but our needs and aspirations are different now, and they will change over time.

With things like appraisal coming in, and allowing us all an annual review of whatever furrow we are ploughing, and asking ourselves the question 'Is it the right one?' then we may see a more mobile and fluid way of employing the GP workforce emerge.

If we can give you any hint it is to wear whatever roles you have lightly, and not to become so stuck in one that you cannot change or modify it later. Times change and we change with them. GP partnerships and other GP employers need to recognise and allow for this.

Places and tasks GPs may become involved in

GP–patient consultations	Commissioning	Legal work
Surgery	Quality control	Medical defence organisations
Walk-in centre	Appraisal and revalidation	Other medico-legal work
Out-of-hours	Medical directors	Expert witness
Running a practice, in-house quality improvement	Responsible officers	Advisory roles
Academic jobs	Substance misuse	Public health
Postgraduate GP training	Prison work	Capacity assessments for benefits (e.g. employment and support allowances)
Undergraduate teaching	Homelessness	
Research	Ship doctor	
Medical politics	Army doctor	
Local medical committee	Sports doctor	Medical journalism and writing
British Medical Association	Occupational health	
RCGP	Health screening	Personal medical services
GPwSI	Recreational medicals	Life insurance medicals
Side specialties	Benefits examiner	
Private GP	Other special projects	

Chapter **5**

Levels of medical effectiveness

Peter Davies

As a doctor you will be working at many levels. It is useful for us to define these so that we are clear about which level we are working at, as the tasks and rules alter at each level of the game.

- Doctor – patient consultation
- Doctor – partnership/local colleagues
- Doctor – local area
- Doctor – region
- Doctor – national

As a doctor you will be involved at some or all of these levels. The question for you as a new GP is which levels are relevant to you now and which levels may become relevant to you in the future.

DOCTOR – PATIENT CONSULTATION

I hope you are good at this; I hope we would not let you off the vocational training scheme if you were not good at this. **If you want any credibility at all as a doctor you had better be good at this**. For young GPs, time spent getting to know your new patients is time well spent, and this will save you much effort in future years. The doctor–patient consultation is the basic unit of all medical practice in primary and secondary care. If you are not effective at this then it is unlikely that your career will flourish, and the sooner you move to something else the better for you and your patients.

This level of medicine is so fundamental that all else builds on the basis of this. It has **an intrinsic value and dignity in its own right**, and for many doctors it is the be-all and end-all of medicine – for them it is what medicine is all about. It should not be discounted or devalued if a doctor moves to work at other levels.

Indeed, the work done at the other levels should be justified by the fact that it makes it easier for colleagues to complete their work at this level, on what is the core task of medicine – namely, treating patients who are ill. The superstructure of the NHS must exist to make it easier for doctors and other clinicians to treat their patients. If it does not help, it is totally unjustified and non-contributory bureaucracy and should be challenged strongly, until it is scrapped. Leadership is only justified to the extent that it helps others to do their jobs better.

The consultation is so important that we consider aspects of it much further in Chapter 13, regarding dealing with isolation and clinical uncertainty, and Chapter 14, regarding adapting consultation skills to the world of actual general practice.

DOCTOR – PARTNERSHIP/LOCAL COLLEAGUES

This is the next important level of medical effectiveness. Indeed, if you are successful at this level then you are likely to work in an effective practice and have an enjoyable career. Your immediate colleagues in practice are probably either your greatest joy or your greatest sorrow.

You will also have a network of more distant colleagues such as health visitors, district nurses and the local hospital staff. These people are rather a given in a local NHS set up and they do not have as much immediate impact on your life as your direct practice colleagues. However, you should get to know them and develop good relationships with them. The local network and culture of a practice is what will make your time there either enjoyable or awful.

Sir Winston Churchill once commented that 'we make our buildings and they in turn make us'. In practices we make our medical 'house' and we can either build it well in collaboration with others or we can tear it down in a demolition derby, leaving dilapidated services and dilapidated doctors in its wake.

The role of **senior partners** in the maintenance of the practice as a medical home is underappreciated. In my own practice we have just lost our senior partner Dr Aiyappa and we are now reforming as a practice team. A shelter and stabilising force has gone, and we are now aware of how much he helped us all by holding things together.

Some practices have a **managing or 'lead' partner**, or a **practice chairman**, who consciously acts as the coordinator and leader of the practice. In the old days such roles used to go by default to the senior partner – which was sometimes great and sometimes a recipe for disaster. There is a lot to be said for having a lead partner for the practice, someone who consciously accepts this role and who has specific time protected for this vital function. For convenience in this chapter I use 'senior partner' to also signify the lead partner.

For young GPs, if you can find a well-run practice with a benign senior partner, then you may well have found a good place to stay. Make sure the senior partner has sufficient longevity that you'll benefit from his experience for a few years before he retires.

Make a distinction between **a senior partner** and **an old partner**. A proper senior partner is one of the best GP characters you will ever meet – wise, tolerant, has seen most things, has a good knowledge of people and has some tolerance for their weaknesses and absurdities. An old partner may well be presented as the senior partner but his or her seniority merely consists of the passage of time and not the accumulation of wisdom and perspective. One of the best ways of spotting a really good senior partner is that they have a concern to make sure their handover of skills and knowledge is complete before they retire. They are looking to bring new people through, not to protect their status. I can think of two particularly good examples of the type I have met personally; they both showed their concern for the future by launching new building projects that meant new premises were being constructed in their last few years of work – new premises that they knew they would not personally get to enjoy for long. They launched the projects to provide continuity and opportunity for their younger colleagues, and they led and tolerated the disruption to routine work that building work causes.

Partnership dynamics are endlessly fascinating, and it takes a lifetime to get very good at them, by which time you retire. In most partnerships there is some degree of tolerance needed, as we all have our bad points. When partnerships work well we tend to overlook each other's faults and when they don't we tend to give each other rather too much feedback.

Partnership relationships are odd and very intense. You may meet a charming, intelligent GP from a nearby practice and you may think the practice is lucky to have him or her. However, in the practice their reputation may be mud and their relationships poor. As a GP it pays to make sure that your internal partnership relationships are secure before courting the outside world . . . unless you are actually signalling that you want a move.

Partners and partnerships differ significantly in their speed and adaptability for change. As a new GP you will probably not know how well or badly you handle change. I have seen very intelligent GP innovators be asked to leave their practice because they got too far ahead of their partners; the partners then make all the changes suggested, but over several years of implementation rather than the milliseconds it took for the quick-thinking innovator to see what needed doing.

I have seen laggards delay development of a practice by many years, even when the other partners want to make an improvement. As a young GP I made the mistake of joining a practice where the older partner was very resistant to change. I was far too much an innovator to spend long in his company, and when I woke up I moved away.

As GPs our relationship to our partnership alters over time. What seems an object of desire in your early career may become a hindrance later on. Few of us know whether we are innovators, consolidators or laggards, and perhaps if we did we might appoint one another as such. For example, a practice may have many innovators in it at one time (like attracts like), and that practice may work, or it may fail, as it has too many ideas in it as once, and it has too few completers and consolidators. Some practices have too many consolidators and laggards and need an innovator to join them, but they need to realise that the dynamic new partner will cause them trouble, and they may not be able to contain him or her. I have a feeling that some GPs should be appointed as innovators, for a short term only, to complete an improvement task and to then move on, as they are unlikely to be happy staying in one place for too long. I also have a feeling that practices should learn to value innovators but learn to release them with good grace when they have completed their task. Likewise, some of the consolidators and laggards should be appointed for long time periods to keep services ticking over, without making too much change. They may not be quick thinkers but they will get the work done.

Knowing where you stand in relation to change is a useful ability for any GP, younger or older, and this will help you find a practice that matches you.

Finally, remember that few jobs expect you to remain in one post at one task for 30–40 years of your life. General practice is unusual among modern British jobs in its potential to be so long-lasting, in one role, in one place. This is either the great strength of GPs or a weakness in our job structure. Increasingly it is becoming common for GP partners to move between practices, or between roles. The old days when a partner who moved was assumed to be a bit odd or flawed (and the partnership he was leaving fine and well organised) have now largely gone. If you are moving jobs you will be asked by the new practice why you are leaving the old one, but there is a much greater acceptance that often it is better for a GP to move away from where he or she is a poor fit to a place where they are a better match with the practice. Also, the new practice may well want some past experience rather than a raw recruit straight off the vocational training scheme.

Whatever sort of GP you are, relating well to your immediate practice colleagues is an effective and enjoyable way of working.

DOCTOR – LOCAL AREA

At some stage all GPs realise that their work and their practice are part of a local area, a local medical ecosystem, and that there is a significant amount of work that needs doing at this level of organisation. Indeed, the commissioning process is forcing GPs to look at what contribution they make to their local area and its activity patterns and finances. The days of GPs being able to hide behind the door of their consulting room or within their own practice are now going, and I think this is actually an improvement to be welcomed. It will naturally bring us into a wider circle of people and activities and therefore increase our opportunities for learning. It will also break down some of the parochialism of practices, and we may come to realise that St Elsewhere's and St Hereabout's can learn a bit from each other.

Some GPs love this aspect of their work, and some GPs want to avoid this level of work. Some are genuinely too busy for this work, but often busyness is an excuse to disguise other priorities and values. Some GPs are just too shy or too scared to join in debate at this level of activity. They prefer the security of their consulting room and their well-known partners.

However, there are important aspects of the medical ecosystem that are put in place at the local area level. For example, the path links system delivering the lab results from your local hospital has not just happened: people drawn from the hospital, primary care and health informatics will have made it happen.

The main roles that GPs take up in their local area involve one of the following:
- the primary care trust
- the nascent commissioning consortia
- the local medical committee
- work as a GP trainer or as a local training programme director
- work as an appraiser or as appraisal lead
- quality assurance work, management of performance issues, medical director
- RCGP local faculty.

What you tend to find is that GPs who see the importance of the area network and want to move to work on their job rather than in their job tend to be a small and readily recognisable proportion of the total GP population. These sorts of roles rapidly attract 'the usual suspects' and 'the committee types'. These usual suspects are either the dynamic and far-sighted local leaders of the NHS or those who have a boring home life and too few hobbies and who are a bit atypical of 'ordinary coalface GPs.' Local knowledge will help you to know which characterisation here is accurate.

Needless to say, the authors of this book are all distinctly part of the usual suspects group, and we regard it as an interesting and entertaining part of our careers, and as a chance to meet interesting people and work on improving how the local medical ecosystem works. For us, our career as GPs would be poorer if we did not join in at this level.

My senior partner, who works full time in clinical practice, says I am too interested at this level and he describes me as 'a dilettante GP'. I would say that I have an interesting portfolio of roles. We enjoy the discussion.

The number of roles open to GPs who want to work at this level is expanding significantly. They do take time and energy, and they take time away from direct clinical care and practice contribution. There is a balance to strike between the interest of these roles and the need to actually keep enough GPs around in the surgeries to provide good enough primary care access.

Some young GPs are worried that there will not be enough jobs to go round. Seeing the expansion of roles at this level makes me wonder if there will actually be enough GPs in the country to fulfil them all and to keep a decent primary care service going (as we saw in Chapter 4).

For younger GPs, these roles are probably best sought after a few years of experience in practice. However, if you want to move towards these roles, then you can make preliminary moves (e.g. attend a few local medical committee meetings, contact the training programme director and ask about training opportunities and so forth) earlier rather than later. All of us on these various boards and committees could use some extra help and some new blood. Approach us and you will find most are keen to help and develop our younger colleagues.

DOCTOR – REGION

In the NHS the regional level used to be very important. It still is for some things, but the strategic health authorities are due to be abolished in 2013. This will then leave a gap in which we will discover what they actually did.

Most GPs could live happily in ignorance of what their local strategic health authority was doing. However, we should be careful about such ignorance. For instance, in March 2011 in Yorkshire an odd consultation came out from the strategic health authority regarding paediatrics and the role of GPs in the care of children. As a regional body, the local faculty of the RCGP responded strongly to the consultation, pointing out the many flaws and false assumptions in its questions.

It is not clear what the regional tier of the NHS will become, but some primary care involvement will be needed at that level.

Most university departments of general practice work at a regional or area level, and with the increasing importance of primary care as an avenue for undergraduate teaching, they have many opening to those GPs willing to learn teaching skills. If, as a young GP, this is where you see your career going, then it is worth getting into a university role and getting your higher degree out of the way sooner rather than later.

DOCTOR – NATIONAL

This level is fascinating and horrifying in equal measure. Doctors here tend to be experienced and to have had prior experience in local area roles. They tend to work as part of the RCGP Council or one of its special interest groups. Alternatively, they are on the General Practitioners Committee. Some others are involved as advisers on Department of Health (DH) projects or as part of the National Institute for Health and Clinical Excellence, the National Patient Safety Agency or the NHS Connecting for Health. When you meet people who work at this level you will become aware that they have a perspective and insight that GPs who stay in their consulting rooms do not. They tend to be discrete, tactful, well-informed and good negotiators.

At this level decisions are made that shift whole frames of reference for our daily work in our consulting rooms (e.g. the impact of the new General Medical Services contract (GMS2), which came into force in 2004).

Indeed, the current 'problem' of 'First5® GPs' has emerged since the 2004 contract. Before that, newly trained GPs were just as naïve as they are now, but at least they all could find GP partnerships and live out their bewilderment with colleagues on a basis of more or less equality. For practices it made more sense to have a partner than a salaried employee. Under the new contract there is a temptation for practices to employ salaried staff rather than partners. Now there are differences emerging between the various groups in the profession such as salaried, partners and freelancers. The authors hope we will remain as a united specialty and that we will sort these differences out.

Work at this level often seems remote from the concerns of the day-to-day work of a GP in the consulting room. Yet if it goes wrong the consequences are disastrous, for doctors and for patients, and often for the DH too. Personally, I think the GMS2 contract was a mistake for the DH, the GPs and the patients. I am looking forward to GMS3 as soon as we can get up momentum in the profession and the government for an improved GP contract that puts the right incentives back into the clinical work in our surgeries.

If you want an example of good work at this level then try reading the RCGP working party report called *The Future General Practitioner*. I read *The Future General Practitioner* about 7 years ago, just out of curiosity, and realised that the whole of my career has been played out in the frames of reference laid down in this book. This book envisaged things in 1973 that at the time were hardly even considered but which are now routine. *The Future General Practitioner* has only just had all its recommendations implemented, but its influence over the whole of general practice education, performance management and continuing professional development cannot be understated.

There is huge power and influence being wielded at this level and it is fascinating and worthwhile work to become part of this. It is all the more powerful for not being 'immediately obvious' or 'directly relevant to your day in the surgery'.

MOVING UP THE LEVELS

As you move up the levels you will notice an increasing change:
- from individual clinical practice towards management of clinical practice

- from dealing with the individual patient towards dealing with many
- from one high-quality consultation towards enough reasonable quality consultations
- from individual excellence towards reasonably reliable systems
- from quality to quantity
- from the consultation to the appointment system
- from my work to the surgery's work
- from the specific to the more abstract
- from the one to the many
- from individual patients to population-based medicine/public health
- from deontological to utilitarian ethics
- from working in the job to working on the job.

The work at the higher levels depends on and grows from the work at the lower levels. The lower levels are lower in terms of being more foundational, not in terms of being inferior in value. The key thing for a GP of any age to know is where he or she stands on these levels and at what level he or she works most effectively – the GP can then adjust his or her job to work at the level at which he or she is most effective.

As a profession we have been slow to acknowledge these levels and the different skills needed at each of them. We have also been slow to acknowledge that, as GPs, we change and develop over time and that our job plans need to alter and adapt to this. We hope that as a new GP you will find this description of levels of medical effectiveness a useful map as you make your way through general practice.

Chapter **6**

How to find a job

Peter Davies and Lindsay Moran

HOW TO FIND A JOB AS A GP

> *When all that is available is nothing, then anything may mistakenly come to be seen as something useful.*

Many new GPs are worried that they will not be able to find a job. Who wants a freshly trained doctor with limited experience when there are plenty of more qualified doctors out there? The authors are well acquainted with this recent feeling, but, rather than not finding work, it is more likely that the problem you will face is the opposite. You certainly should be able to find a job in the current climate, but it may not be exactly what you want or where you want it. **The danger for young GPs is not that they end up underemployed, but that they end up overemployed somewhere they don't want to be.**

It would be lovely to think that we will all find our ideal job, at an early stage of our careers, and work away at it with skill and purpose for many years to come. Actually the job of a GP has never really been like that. It may take a few goes to land yourself in the right practice, with compatible partners and plus or minus a portfolio you are proud of. It seems to be inherently built into the minds of young GPs that partnerships are the Holy Grail we all strive for, and that may be the case for many, but there is no need to rush. It is not only about reaching the destination but also about making sure you enjoy the experience of the journey along the way.

SOME GENERAL COMMENTS ABOUT JOBS

1. **Jobs are an unstable balance across satisfaction, salary and support**. My friend Adrian Kenny (now a GP in Australia) usefully described this to me. We all make trade-offs between these three things, and value certain aspects more highly at certain times of our careers. It is worth assessing any job under these three headings, and becoming conscious of which aspects of the triangle you value more or less. As a general rule, the less support and the less satisfaction a job has the more the employer has to pay to get it done. Most medical jobs should score well on satisfaction and interest. However, the quality of support is often what determines whether the job is enjoyable or not. Salary levels in medicine are usually reasonable.

2. **We very rarely know our goal when we enter a jobs market**. Often getting a job at all seems like a good first move. If you are lucky it is. Often this strategy garners experience, but results in later moves. John Kay describes how our goals (personal or corporate) are often achieved **obliquely**.[1] We do not fully know where we are starting from, we do not know fully where we want to get to, and so we have to make a few moves towards where we think we want to be, but these moves are often tentative and uncertain. He suggests that our life goals and purposes are often not fully defined in the early stages of a journey. For new GPs setting out into practice this is worth bearing in mind – you may not know clearly where you want to get to. Even those who apparently have a clear goal may end up revising it.

3. **Jobs are ultimately about economics** – about earning money enough to keep you and families and partners in the style to which you and they want to become accustomed. It is nice if your job has purpose and vision and meets your needs for higher realisation, but the starting point is lower down **Maslow's hierarchy** and is about securing food, warmth and shelter in the first instance.

4. **'Take this job and shove it'**. Before launching this tirade at your boss, remember that you have a basic need to put food on the table, which might temper your attitude to your job, at least for a short while. Many of our patients are putting up with worse jobs for a lot longer than we have to. Churchill once stated that many of us are 'humdrum people living ordinary lives of quiet desperation'. You may be one of them for a while.

5. **Do not overvalue a job**. Sad as this sounds, if you die your colleagues will miss you, send flowers to your funeral, but then they will get on with the work. They will have extra work to cover for a while, but you will be replaceable. As I write this I am thinking of a highly respected Yorkshire GP who died at a young age from a brain tumour. She contributed a lot to her family, her practice and GP education. She was talking with a senior colleague about perspective and the things that really mattered – family, doing the right

thing –and she agreed with him that a lot of what *exercises us relating to NHS management* is an irrelevant game. We do well to keep our **work–life balance** under review throughout our careers.

6. **Children change everything**. The combination of establishing a career and having children is a lot of things to do at once, particularly for female GPs. And this is before you factor in the effects of sleep deprivation and the general disruption caused by children – even the good ones. Children change what you think, and how you think, and that is in the lucid moments when you have caught up with your sleep enough to think.

7. **For most jobs movement is expected**. Few people now have jobs for life, and indeed the feeling is that a job should not be for life now. Long-term jobs may be seen as leading to complacency, outdated and obsolete skills, boredom, burnout and lack of growth and challenge. Most people seem to need a new challenge every so often. The phenomenon of long-serving GPs holding down their jobs for 20–30 years is unusual in the current employment climate.

8. **Job-hunting is like courtship rather than competition**. There are some jobs for which you are a good fit, and some for which you are not suited. Looking back on my career I can think of many occasions when I have not got a job, and only later realised how lucky it was that I did not get it. Equally, I have regretted some jobs that I have taken.

WHERE TO FIND A GP JOB

There are lots of places to find a GP job, you just have to look.

- Websites:
  - NHS Jobs (www.jobs.nhs.uk)
  - Doctors.net.uk (www.doctors.net.uk)
  - GP Jobs (http://jobs.gponline.com)
  - some local GP specialty training scheme websites host job adverts
  - your favourite search engine – type in 'GP jobs'.
- Magazines and publications:
  - *BMJ Careers*
  - *GP* (borrow it from the surgery coffee room if you are in the surgery)
  - *Pulse* (same as above).
- Contacting the surgery directly:
  - go to the NHS Choices website (www.nhs.uk), type in your postcode, and search for surgeries around your locality. Then call the surgery and speak to the practice manager. It's easier (and cheaper) to get their email address to send them your CV electronically rather than posting it.
- Organisations:
  - your local medical committee group may have a job section

- local RCGP faculty
- local deanery.
- Job agencies:
  - an easy way of picking up extra work, but remember, they'll be taking their cut for your work too.
- Word of mouth:
  - a bit like being on the dating scene – make it be known to all that you're available and to let you know if any practice wants you to hook up!

YOUR CURRICULUM VITAE

Before looking for your dream job, you might want to spice up your CV to sell yourself. It is the balance between giving enough information and not giving your future employer a novel that puts them soundly off to sleep. For each job you go for you may wish to alter your CV. For a locum job it is preferable to try to keep your CV to two sides of an A4 sheet of paper. Your other jobs, perhaps an academic post or a partnership where they are wanting you to demonstrate what you can bring to the table, you may wish to be more inclusive about your past experiences and achievements.

The template given here to start you off may be more comprehensive than you need, but apply that which is relevant.

Dr New GP

Personal details
Address: 1 The Big Apartment, Down the Street, in the Town.
GMC No:
Medical Indemnity No:
Contact telephone:
Email:

Possible additional information includes nationality, date of birth, latest Criminal Records Bureau check, driving licence, smartcard number, personal photo. While there is no need to state these, it may satisfy the curiosity of your new employer.

Career statement
What drives you as a doctor? What are your positive attributes that will make you attractive to this new employer? What experience do you have that will complement their practice? How do you fit into a team? What are your short-term and long-term career goals?

Tailor this statement to fit with the job that you are applying for. You can mention how long you have lived in the area and that you are happy and settled (if this is the case).

Education and qualifications
Diplomas:
Professional memberships:
(i.e. membership to any professional bodies such as the RCGP, international bodies, committee participation)
Primary medical qualification:

Employment history
Include all recent jobs and explain any career gaps.

Current commitments
What skills do you currently have in your present employment? You can list them under the headings of:
Clinical skills and experience
Educational skills
Management and leadership skills.
It can also be useful to mention your notice period.

Computer experience
Which GP computer systems are you proficient at? Are your general computing skills acceptable?

Publications
If relevant, this may be of benefit and interest to your employer.

Personal interests and recreation
Provide a short paragraph on who you are and what you like doing.

Referees
Ideally two, a maximum of three should be provided. Preferably this would include a clinical colleague from your most recent job. You should also tailor your referees to the post you are applying for, i.e. if you are applying for an academic or teaching post, then a referee with experience of supervising you in this field would be helpful. When selecting a referee, remember to notify them first. Ideally this person should have known you for more than a year.

Many CVs look very similar. Dr Young Hopeful, MBChB, MRCGP, looks like all the others on paper. The CV needs to tell employers who and what you are about. Reading CVs, we can spot who sends their CV by email to each practice that is advertising this week. For example, if you live in Hampshire and are applying to a practice in Yorkshire, please tweak your CV or the covering letter to say why you want to make this move. Otherwise we may guess that you do not really want to move. If, however, you went to the University of Southampton and now want to return to Yorkshire to be closer to family . . . well, we'll see if we can help you.

High-quality paper and good printing does still make a good impression. It makes you look high quality, and certainly of higher quality than routine white A4 paper, but then again, email is the choice for many doctors these days too.

A good covering letter saying where you heard about the vacancy and why it appeals to you is very useful and can put you ahead of your competition.

PRELIMINARY VISITS

The candidates who really want a job will send in a well-presented CV soon after the advert appears (within a week). They will then follow up with phone calls to the practice managers and one or more partners.

Visiting the practice beforehand is a good move. It shows interest and initiative. It makes you a person, not just a name on a CV. It allows you to assess the mood of a practice, and the practice to assess you. Much basic information exchange can happen, and you can see rapidly if there is a match or mismatch between you and the practice. It shows interest and politeness, and you trying to find out about what kind of practice it is, what it needs, and what you can bring to it. This process will ensure that you become more than a name on a pile of CVs and become a character in whom the partnership will take an interest.

While asking the practice directly you will also be making local enquiries to discover more about the practice and how it is regarded locally, and find out whether it is the kind of place where they would want to work. By the time of any interview such candidates will already know a lot about the practice. One particular tip is to enquire at the local pharmacies about relations with the practice of interest.

Because all GPs now have MRCGP it is now a less useful discriminator than it used to be. Hence, young GPs now need to establish themselves as people and so get themselves onto the shortlist.

The practice reciprocally may discover a lot about the applicant. Your training programme director is often asked informally about you, as may be consultants you have worked for. One of the pleasures of receiving CVs is that it often gives employers a chance to have a phone call to catch up with an old mate they knew years ago. They may even discuss the candidate.

A matching game is going on both ways, seeing whether the employers want you and whether you want them.

The more you can show employers what you bring and how you could help them with the development of their practice, the more chance you have of getting the job. Interest, politeness, enthusiasm, ability – the more you show an employer these qualities the more interested in you they will become.

INTERVIEWS

In a job appointment process both sides are **trying to find out about the other**. The applicant is fearful, and a bit needy and wondering if they can get the job, and will enjoy it if they do. The appointers are also a bit needy – they need a new colleague, and want someone who they will like, who the staff and patients will like, and who will not disrupt the practice unnecessarily. They want someone whose clinical practice they can respect – they do not want to have to review all your decisions! You may think jobs are allocated on the basis of qualifications and such like. In practice they largely go on the basis of **perceived competence, your willingness for work and likeability**. Also, although officially all jobs are open to all without sex bias, you can quickly work out in most practices if they want or need a man or woman as the next member of the team.

Some practices are looking for **specific extra skills**, or a willingness to take on certain roles such as GP training. As an applicant you should know whether this is something you want to do or not. Be honest: if your mindset or skill set is not right for a particular job, well that is best discovered in preliminary discussions rather than at interview or after appointment. At the end of the process the practice and the new doctor want to **match each other well**. If you can **work out what the practice needs**, and then whether and how you can meet that need then you have a good chance of getting the job. If you are not the solution to their problems then the job is not for you – move on and let another doctor take it.

Although interviews are officially about finding out about the applicant, the panel of doctors making the decision may not know each other very well. They may not know exactly what they are looking for, or they may each be looking for different things in an applicant. The interview process may bring out partnership differences. The panel may appear cohesive and terrifying to the applicant but they may actually be a bit of a rabble. A well-organised interview panel will be well structured, the partners will have defined what they are looking for beforehand, and they will be using structured questions to learn about the applicants.

Although those interviewing you should all have read your CV carefully, do not assume they have done so. They are busy people with many things to read, and they may only have skimmed or glanced at the CV you have so carefully prepared. You may well be asked to restate basic details that are clearly stated in your CV.

It is useful to show that you have found out about the practice you have applied to. **If you can convince the partners that you know something about their work, respect it, and have a good reason for wanting to join them in it then you will go a long way towards getting the job you want.** Local knowledge, doing locums in an area, speaking to your trainers and other local colleagues (e.g. local medical committee secretary, local consultants), or checking their practice website, NHS Choices or www.gpcontract.co.uk for practice perform-ance data may give you additional useful information about whether to apply to the practice or not.

A FEW TIPS FOR THE INTERVIEW
- Dress smart
- Talk about your positive qualities
- Be inquisitive about the practice
- Be clear why you want this job

Things to ask before or at the interview
Remember, this is like the dating game: you want them to like you and you need to like them.
- What is the salary?
- Any flexibility in hours, sessions (i.e. to work around childcare or other work commitments)?
- Do you offer the British Medical Association (BMA) model contract? (Even if the answer is yes, it's worthwhile checking it with the association.)
- What gets discussed at practice meetings and will you be invited if salaried?
- What are the surgery times, visits, on-call and extended hours commitments? Also, what administration time is there?
- Are they looking for anything in particular (i.e. a future GP trainer)?
- What would be your Quality and Outcomes Framework responsibilities?
- Is the practice personal medical services or general medical services?
- Will there be any opportunity of a future partnership?
- Why is there a vacancy now?
- If it is a split practice, where would the majority of clinical sessions be?
- Do you get sick leave/maternity leave and what is your holiday entitlement?

Things to ask specifically at a partnership job interview
This is a little beyond dating. You need to assess this from a 'would I marry you?' perspective now.
- Why is there a partnership vacancy now?
- How many partners are there currently and what is the WTE (working time equivalent) of those partners? Also, what is the male : female ratio?

- Are there any non-medical partners?
- Is there parity (the time taken to receive full partner pay) in the business and what is the time to parity? Can you buy in if needed?
- Is there a hierarchy system in place?
- What type of partner are they looking for? Any specialist skills needed?
- What lead are they looking for in their new partner?
- Do they own the building?
- What is their capital?
- What is the Quality and Outcomes Framework achievement?
- What are the sessional commitments for this partnership? Is there any flexibility to this?
- Do they have extended hours?
- Does the job include staff appraisals?
- Is it a training practice? If so, is the training grant shared out? This also applies to GPwSI (GP with a special interest) payments.
- How much do the partners get paid (gross and net)?
- What are the practice expenses?
- What is the organisational structure?
- What is your sick leave/maternity leave entitlement and is there locum cover for this?
- Are they amenable to you taking a sabbatical?
- Be sure you also know how the partnership agreement can be terminated.

It is advisable that once you enter into serious negotiations with a practice you get an accountant to look over their books for the last 3 years to make sure there are no skeletons lurking in any closets. You should also spend time sitting with the practice accountant.

NEGOTIATING YOUR SALARY

You've just finished your training, a kind practice offers you a job despite your gross lack of experience ... everything looks good, until they present a substandard salary offer to you. You're terrified to negotiate unless they decide they don't want you and will offer the job instead to another inexperienced GP who doesn't have the bottle to argue.

Well, generally speaking, if you think the offer isn't good enough, make sure you negotiate. You have skills that they want and, like the L'Oréal advert says, you're worth it! There is also information available about the average salary available in your area, from the BMA.

- You can negotiate your salary (I would like £70 000, not £65 000, for those eight sessions).

- You can ask for your General Medical Council registration and indemnity insurance to be included in the contract (although you may not get it).
- Continuing professional development time can be negotiated (although this is specified in the BMA model contract).
- Get it in writing when your pay review will be and what the increment is likely to be.
- Private work (i.e. insurance reports) are also negotiable.

Contractually, general medical services practices should offer you the BMA model contract, whereas personal medical services practices have no obligation to do so. If you work for a private company, they can do whatever they please!

THE GP JOBS MARKET

Some historical perspective is useful here. Many years ago (about 1930–60) GP partners exploited younger GPs, employing them as 'assistants' or as 'assistant with a view to partnership'. This view was a long view and rarely honoured. The younger GPs were of course paid far less, and the partner was raking off the extra profits. This kind of scenario is well described in *The Citadel* by AJ Cronin.[2]

Things moved on, and under **the 1966 and 1990 GP contracts** it became advantageous to practices to take on partners rather than salaried doctors. Each new partner brought with them a large 'basic practice allowance'. So we ended up with a profession with a **flat hierarchy** in which everyone was a partner or a GP trainee (registrar). This had many merits, but it also had some absurdities in that it was clear that some GP partners either were, or should be, a lot more equal than others. The partnership system was on the whole fair. The worst aspect was '3 years till parity' (of profit share), but at least everyone was at a basic level and in the same system.

Looking **outside medicine**, other professions such as law and accountancy have far more complex partnership structures and levels than we do. It is very unlikely that any lawyer would expect to move into a partnership just on the basis of having gained their basic practising certificate. Most lawyers have to put in many years of work at lower levels of their law firms before they even reach a junior partnership. Many never reach partnership.

For GP partnerships the **new General Medical Services contract** in 2004 changed everything. It rejuvenated many partnerships, and financial rewards increased. However, under the new arrangements it has become expedient for practices to take on salaried doctors, and not admit them into the partnership. Practices have absolute discretion on whether to take on partners or salaried doctors, or any other staff for that matter. Now most practices are taking on doctors on a salary for a period (6–24 months) before considering partnership. We are almost back to the 'assistant with view' days of many years ago.

Some practices are being sensible and using a salaried period to get to know a new doctor and see if they fit into their partnership. This is beneficial for both parties, as getting the wrong partner or being the wrong partner is no fun for either side.

Sadly, many practices are being short-sighted and venial, preferring to churn through many salaried doctors, rather than to develop and induct them into the partnership. Peter has seen many intelligent younger GPs being forced away by big, well-organised practices in which the partners have decided not to be generous with the partnership. The short-sightedness comes that the partnership leaders are the partners, and that salaried GPs tend not to be the practice leaders. If as a specialty and as GP partnerships we are not bringing our younger colleagues through into the partnerships and leadership, then we are steadily destroying our own organisations.

Anyway, the outcome of all this history is that as a new GP currently you will find yourself choosing between different types of employment option, all of which have strengths and weaknesses.

Overall, all of the options have their strengths and weaknesses, but generally there is a great demand for GPs in the job market and no doubt you will find a job to suit your needs. The need for a generalist is always in demand.

REFERENCES

1 Kay JA. *Obliquity: why our goals are best achieved indirectly.* London: Profile Books; 2010.
2 Cronin AJ. *The Citadel.* Boston: Little, Brown and Co; 1937.

A Partnerships

Peter Davies, with input from Lindsay Moran

Pros	Cons
More money (it is to be hoped!)	Time-consuming
Business skills	Less flexible
Reliability	Costly to buy into
Stability	
Continuity	
Ownership	

Partnership has many benefits: stability, reliability, support and continuity of patients and colleagues. Often financially rewarding (but not always – many practices earn poorly), the average full-time partner these days is said to earn around £110 000 a year. Partnership provides a base and a medical home to the doctor. It gets your name on the door and on the headed notepaper. It earns you a say in discussions and in the organisation of the practice. It gives you a **sense of ownership of your work** – as a partner you never 'just work here'.

Partnerships are usually intended to be permanent, and to last several years, and probably until retirement. They are not to be entered into if you plan to go travelling round the world for 6 months next year. Get your travelling done and out of the way, and then see what partnerships are on offer once you have settled. You need to decide that you like the practice and that you like the area and want to make your home there.

The disadvantages of partnership are similar to the advantages. **Ownership implies responsibility**, and owning the work of the practice, and not just the direct clinical work. You may have to deal with awkward staff. You have to keep accounts. You have to keep the staff and premises intact and organised. You have to attend the practice meetings.

To some, all this may seem daunting, but actually in well-organised practices the practice manager has most of the necessary processes in place. If you are lucky, the senior (or management lead) partner has most of the business sorted out before you join. You can then take some time to learn as you go. If we are honest, very few partners arrive knowing everything about a business and most of us need help from older colleagues to learn this side of the business. The

Radcliffe 'Making Sense' series of books (such as *Making Sense of the Red Book*) were very important to us when we were starting. The modern equivalent is Mike Gilbert's book *Managing Money for General Practitioners: 2*.[1]

What partners are looking for is a realisation that the work of the partnership is about more than the direct clinical work. These days if you give off signals that you 'just want to see patients' then expect to be offered a salaried post, not a partnership. Partners are in a partnership 'with a view to profit' and they make this by means of their medical work.

You need to build up a capital stake in the workings of the practice. This is working capital in the business, and/or a stake in the premises. This will involve raising funds, usually from the bank, unless you have a rich family member who will set you up. Most practices will have capital accounts of between £20 000 and £40 000 per GP. If the partners own the building their capital accounts will be about £150 000–£300 000, reflecting the stake in the building. This looks like a lot of money, but remember that the notional rent covers the payments on a business loan used to buy a share of the building. Generally GPs who own their own premises earn more than those in rented premises. If you get a chance to buy into an owner-occupied GP building it is usually a good move to take the chance (but, as always, check with the accountant first).

Some partners build up their stake in the business by reducing their drawings, so leaving additional money in the practice account. This reduces your personal cash flow for a while, but it can save you the need to borrow money. You need to think of your partnership as an asset to yourself that will give you a good return in the long term. The short-term problem of raising a capital sum is a temporary local difficulty that you will look back on in later years and wonder why you worried about it so much when you started.

Some practices have a parity system in place. This system means younger partners earn a lower share of the profits in each of their early years in the practice, till they reach an equity stake in the partnership. This was something that used to be commonplace, but it is a rare arrangement nowadays. The old arrangement was usually '3 years till parity'. This was not too bad, as you were joining a profitable business that would give you good earnings over time, a secure medical home and some decent colleagues. Never allow temporary current difficulties to blind you to the likely unfolding of events over the next 5–20 years.

As a partner you are expected to be loyal to the practice, and not to move away from it. This used to be an almost absolute rule, but now it is more relaxed. GP partners can and do move between practices – indeed, some practices welcome those with experience as a partner elsewhere. If you are moving as a partner, anticipate being asked about why you are moving from one practice to another.

There are two major problems in partnerships that catch out GPs. First, the GPs may not like each other. We spend too much time at work not to like our colleagues. When GPs do fall out, the roots are usually found in disputes about workload allocation and distribution, the on-call rota (less so now, as out-of-hours is usually an external service) and money. Second, partners and partnerships differ in their attitudes towards career development and outside work. This is rarely a problem early in a partnership, but when you have been there for a few years and are looking to take time away from surgeries to learn a new skill (e.g. training) then problems may arise.

Sometimes one of the doctors is just in the wrong place in relation to the partnership. When this happens it is usually better to recognise the problem and then release the doctor to move on. However, like in an amicable divorce the question arises: if you can manage a breakdown so well then why do you need to separate at all?

As a partner you share in the profits of the practice, but you share the losses as well. If profits are rising, all seems to be going well. If profits are falling, then your take-home pay may drop.

Much of your income as a partner comes in later than the work done, so you may have to wait to get all the income you have earned out from the business as a drawing.

Remember that partnership income looks more than the equivalent PAYE salary, but that once you understand the on-costs of employment (employer's National Insurance contributions, employer's pension contribution) then a salary of £77 000 per year is equivalent to a partner's profit share of £100 000 per year.

As I write in mid-2011, GP partnership profits are falling and so your enthusiasm to move into a partnership may not immediately give you a pay rise from your salaried earnings. The way partnership earnings vs. salaried earnings will alter in the future is difficult to predict. In 2000–03 partnership incomes were way down and a risk was emerging that GP partners would quit their partnerships and move into salaried or locum roles. The commercial confidence of locums at that time was huge, and the hassles of partnership were beginning to seem unjustified by the earnings. The 2004 contract did give a big boost to the pay of GP partners, but the initial boost has been whittled away steadily over the last 6 years.

If you want to become a partner, showing an awareness of this business side of a practice will help convince the partners that you understand what you are joining.

REFERENCE

1 Gilbert M. *Managing Money for General Practitioners.* 2nd ed. Oxford: Radcliffe Publishing; 2009.

B Freelance

Lindsay Moran, with input by Hussain Gandhi
and Peter Davies

Pros	Cons
Flexibility	No guaranteed income
Control your own pay	Time-consuming finding work
See a variety of practices	Isolating at times
Good experience	Lack of patient continuity

FREELANCE (SESSIONAL, LOCUM) WORK

A locum GP is *locum tenens* – that is, holding the place of somebody else. As such, the role can be seen as rather like being a substitute in a football match. In the older days a locum GP tended to be just that – a doctor who took the place of another for a short period. Nowadays the work of locum GPs has expanded, and just thinking of 'locums' is rather limited.

There is now a pool of freelance GPs who are available for various roles within general practice. Some have portfolio careers, doing some clinical sessions as a locum and then doing other jobs in other roles. They may think of themselves as freelance workers. For that reason the terms locum, freelance or portfolio doctor are interchangeable with 'non-principals' or 'sessional' doctors, although salaried doctors fit under these descriptions too. Most out-of-hours general practice is done by freelance GPs now. There is a well-developed National Association of Sessional GPs (NASGP), which has started to coordinate activities for freelance GPs. The group of doctors who work as freelance GPs is varied in terms of age and experience and in terms of what work they do. Some are younger (First5®) GPs who are using a spell locuming to experience different practices before choosing to settle down. If you have just moved to a new area, locuming can be a good option to meet other doctors and experience new surgeries. Some are older GPs who for whatever reason have left their partnership behind. Some work as freelance GPs by choice, whereas others are forced into it.

Freelance doctors' clinical commitments to practices vary. Some freelance GPs do a single surgery at short notice, usually because one of the partners is off sick. Such relief can be very welcome to a practice acutely short of doctors.

Some freelance GPs' work is on a fixed-term basis, the most common example here being a 6- or 9-month maternity locum. Many doctors doing such work use it as a springboard to a permanent job, either finding something turns up where they are working or they get a recommendation on to another practice nearby wanting a new doctor.

There are strengths and weaknesses to locum work. From the point of view of a GP partner, short-term locums are an expensive and short-term solution to a (usually unwanted and unanticipated) acute problem such as a partner being off sick. Sadly, the experience of most partners is that the freelance GP sees the patients one day and then the patients return for a review or second opinion from the 'doctor they know' a few days later. However, equally, there are some doctors for whom carrying the whole burden of a practice and continuity of care becomes too much. There may come a stage when you are bored or frustrated, either by your partnership or by your particular pool of patients, and feel a need for more variety in your work. Some doctors just prefer short-term interactions with patients and find long-term management of patients over many years a chore.

Longer-term locums such as maternity locums are often a better proposition. They tend to integrate the doctor into the practice team to get to know the partners and the staff, as well as to know how the place works. They will find out how the local care pathways work. They will carry a share of the practice work outside of the direct clinical contact – such as pathology results, reading letters and so on. The patients get the chance of some continuity, and the freelance GP can get feedback and they can follow up on the patients they have seen.

Therefore, working as a freelance GP can be a good starting point for new GPs. It has its anxieties – 'Will I find enough work?' 'How do things work in this practice?' – yet it can be very rewarding at the same time. You learn a lot about a variety of practices. Each practice operates differently and you learn what you like about particular practices and, more important, what you don't like. However, it can be isolating. You may arrive at a practice to find you are the only doctor working alongside the receptionist! You also find some practices where you do not bump into other clinicians at all. However, generally, most practices are open and friendly and the GPs usually make an effort to meet you. It's a good way of getting to know a few GPs in different practices locally and seeing how different practices operate. If you spread your locuming around different areas it also gives you good experience of working with a range of socio-economic groups.

Given the changes occurring in general practice at present, it is generally quite a good time to find work. More and more there are young female GPs being employed, thus more maternity locums. Several older GPs are considering retiring because of pension changes, and with commissioning diverting many GPs away from clinical practice this again creates a need for locums to fill the clinical work. A lot of freelance GPs worry that they won't get work, and certainly the market differs depending where you are around the country, but generally there is enough locum work to go around. Once you get your name known locally, you'll probably be inundated with offers for work. Because of this it is very important to book your holidays and days off in your diary well in advance.

A friend of mine, after finishing the vocational training scheme, arrived to her first locum session with a box of chocolates to celebrate. This certainly was a popular start!

IS BEING A FREELANCE GP A GOOD ROUTE FOR A NEW GP TO TAKE?

The positives

The answer is yes if you want to see a lot of different practices in action, to control your own diary fully, to control your own workload and income levels, and look towards developing some outside interests. It is a good option for some entrepreneurial GPs who see themselves as a 'medical services company' and then set about marketing their services to various customers, some of whom are fellow GPs and some of whom are in different settings. It can be a good option for some very innovative GPs who struggle to stay contained within a practice.

The other advantage of locum and sessional jobs is that they are finite, and that it is easy to leave them. You are not tied in as a locum.

Some doctors enjoy freelance work because it gives them good control over their work rota and holidays – they simply block out their holiday periods and any wanted days off in advance, and take no bookings on those dates. There is certain straightforwardness to the trading off of income desired against the amount of time you are prepared to work for it. And when you work out the sums for yourself, you tend to make the decisions well for yourself.

Some freelance GPs have a varied portfolio of roles within clinical practice and GP education. The flexibility of locum work may allow them to run this portfolio more smoothly than they could as a GP principal with large and fixed time commitments.

The negatives

The answer is no if you do not like negotiating, if you like a regular settled team, if you want to provide continuity of care, and if you want a regular settled income.

There are some structural weaknesses to locum work. Every patient comes to you as a new case. Your clinical knowledge may be fine, but as my trainer put it to me, 'the specialist works out what disease the patient has, the GP works out what kind of patient has the disease'. That knowledge of patients takes time to develop – you get quicker at it as you grow in experience, but a locum is at a disadvantage compared with a regular doctor. As a result, freelance GPs can become deskilled over time. The lack of interaction in team meetings and access to experienced colleagues for case discussion can present a challenge. To ask new

GPs to take on large surgeries in practices (and maybe areas) they do not know well is potentially risky. It may also be difficult to provide good-quality evidence for appraisal and revalidation.

One of the bugbears in medicine is what Michael Balint described as 'collusion of anonymity'.[1] In this system the patient gets passed from one doctor to another, either within a practice or between GP and hospital, and each doctor does something but none of them really gets a grip on the case. Short-term medicine such as short-term locums, and brief, narrowly focused micro-specialty outpatient appointments, increase the risk of this developing. This recently led Professor Raymond Tallis to lament that doctors risk becoming 'sessional functionaries robotically following guidelines'.[2] Other doctors have worried about the risk of a casualisation of the GP workforce such that, like staff at McDonald's, a GP can be taken out of one place and slotted into another and no one notices any difference. To some extent out-of-hours provider sessions are already done on this basis.

For a GP principal you are thinking of handling a patient over the next 10 years or more. As a locum your time perspective draws in significantly and you will tend to think much more about the current acute illness (days/weeks) than about a long-term (months/years) strategy for a patient. The presence or absence of personal follow-up significantly alters how a doctor approaches a consultation. For short-term locums it makes great sense to do what is needed on the day and to leave the routine work to the regular doctors.

The main feature of sessional GP work, and its main difference from what GP principals do is this issue of time frames, and hence the range of your actions and their effects. Clinically locums are as good as any other group of GPs.

The other main problem for locums is getting good long-term follow-up data about the quality of their work. It is not easy to get good data about established GP principals working for many years in one place. Trying to get a handle on the outcomes of the actions of peripatetic locum doctors is nigh on impossible, unless they are obviously disastrous such as those of Dr Daniel Ubani – the German doctor who administered lethal amounts of pain control to a patient on an out-of-hours shift.

HOW TO FIND WORK AS A LOCUM

It can take a little time before you build up pace to be a full-time locum with a fully booked diary. There are a few ways of finding locum work; this depends really on how much effort you wish to put in and where you choose to seek your work.

1. If you are looking for low maintenance then you can simply sign up with a locum agency and let them do the hard work. The sticking point for me with this is that someone else is then getting a cut of the pay for the work that you do.

2. Put yourself out there. Send your curriculum vitae round all the local GP sur-
    geries (the NHS Choices website (www.nhs.uk) is an excellent site to search
    for local surgeries). Get to know other GPs in your area who are locuming and
    find out via word of mouth who is looking for locums. There may be various
    places locally where jobs are advertised, including the local vocational train-
    ing scheme. Sometimes surgeries will send out their locum requirements to
    a local locum group – it may be worth getting in touch with these.
3. Join a locum chambers. This is a different model entirely. A number of GPs
    get together to form a business model. Usually there is an administration team
    and a small proportion of your salary is used to pay the administration costs
    for this. The chambers will have their set terms and conditions for how they
    operate and have standards that they set for their GPs. This is to set a high
    standard for the practices that will be employing them and to guarantee the
    quality of those working for the chambers.
4. There are a few other companies (Locum Monkey being one example) that
    are free to join as a GP, although they charge the practice to advertise to their
    group of GPs. This is another way to pick up available sessions.

THE PRACTICALITIES

There are a few things to bear in mind before starting your work as a locum. You
need to be registered with your local primary care trust to be on their primary
performers list. It is the primary care trust who will do your Criminal Records
Bureau check and your Criminal Records Bureau check needs to be updated
every 3 years.

You need to maintain your own certificates (i.e. General Medical Council,
indemnity, performers list registration, vaccinations, basic life support certificate
and so forth). Using a calendar to notify you when these are due for renewal can
help prevent last-minute problems.

- Register yourself as self-employed with HM Revenue and Customs (www.
  hmrc.gov.uk/selfemployed/register-selfemp.htm).
- Remember, as self-employed, you will be paid gross pay more likely from
  a practice. This means that normally a year down the line you will receive
  a tax bill. It is always advisable to save a portion of your pay to prepare
  for this. I (Hussain) would recommend 40%, as this should cover any
  tax bill, and leave you with some surplus, depending on how good your
  accountant is.
- Get each job to sign a Pension Form A (www.nhsbsa.nhs.uk/Documents/
  Pensions/GPLocumA.pdf). It is usually easiest to send this form out with
  your invoice.
- At the end of each month complete a Pension Form B (www.nhsbsa.nhs.
  uk/Documents/Pensions/GPLocumB.pdf) and send this off with a cheque

to your local primary care trust office. Usually, most locums pay 6.5% pension. Those earning more than £100 000 may need to pay 7.5%, so contact your primary care trust if your earnings increase beyond this. Keep a record of your pension payments for your tax assessment.

- It is advisable to get a good medical accountant early on. They normally pay for themselves with savings made, and will reduce your own administration time spent on working out tax bills, etc. (i.e. www.GPadvance.com).
- Remember your indemnity covers you for the number of sessions you work for. This is normally classified as a number of sessions per week, i.e. up to four sessions a week. This does raise some leeway. For example, if you work part time at five sessions a week, but with a three month career break planned, then the above cover would be enough. However do note that if you then work over the allotted number of sessions without informing your indemnity company, you may not be suitably covered. If you are in any doubt speak to the membership department at your medical defence organisation.
- Working as a freelance GP, you may want to consider income protection insurance, which can be taken from various providers. As a freelance you are not entitled to 'sick pay', so if you were unable to work, then it raises the question of where will the money come from? Whether you take this is dependent on your own situation and risk aversion. At the very least it is advisable to have a 'savings bunker' to dip into if the need arises.

PAY AND CHARGES

How much should you charge? Essentially you can charge what you like. But what local surgeries will pay will depend on your competition locally.

Some surgeries like to quote their own rates of pay. When I (Lindsay) first started locuming I thought this was an acceptable thing for them to do, until I heard a more experienced freelance GP say how she was astounded that a GP surgery sent her 'their rates' for what they would pay her. She promptly shot them back an email stating 'these are my rates, and my terms and conditions, let me know if you still require my services'. Admittedly it takes some degree of confidence to do this when you are starting out though, and you may find yourself accepting slightly lower rates of pay as a new locum GP until you find your footing.

There are different ways of working out what to charge. I initially started out by charging one rate per session, but I promptly realised that a session could range from 2 to 3 hours, thus that didn't seem too sensible.

It makes more sense to break down your time and perhaps charge an hourly rate. Many GPs will have a minimum rate, i.e. if your hourly rate is £80 and you are asked to do a 2-hour session, you can state that your minimum charge is £210.

Be clear when booking how many patients you will be seeing per hour. If you are happy seeing six patients per hour then state this. Some locums like to include blocks in their surgery and only see five patients per hour. It is good to be clear about the amount of patients to be seen (i.e. 2 hours = 12 patients) because not all surgeries run 10-minute appointments and you'll get quite a shock on arrival if you find out you are expected to see patients at 5-minute intervals.

You would expect that each session you do generates a certain amount of administration. You do not have to charge additional for this, but some locums choose to charge extra for this time. Alternatively, you can include this administration as part of your session, but should you be asked to do additional work on top of this you can charge the practice extra, based on your hourly rate. If you are doing a full day for a practice you can choose to agree to perform paperwork or administration tasks as part of the day package. Some GPs include mileage in their charges, especially if the surgery is beyond a certain travel distance (i.e. 5 miles).

Home visits

Most locums would usually charge per home visit, or if you have agreed to do a full day you can specify two visits. Above this you can charge for extra visits.

It is difficult to quote rates here as from talking to colleagues I know that locum rates do vary across the country and this is usually based on demand. A good place to look for further information on this is the NASGP.

Be clear when stating charges. As you will be self-employed, you are free to set your own rates and this is something to be negotiated with the practices. There is no one set rate that locums charge – indeed, setting one rate is illegal and will fall under the watch of the Office of Fair Trading, should this happen! Rates tend to vary depending on where you are in the country and how much demand there is for locums in the area.

For example, your charges list may look like this:
- Hourly rate – £80
- 2 hours (12 patients) – £210 (minimum charge)
- 2.5 hours (15 patients) – £225 (minimum charge)
- 3 hours (18 patients) – £240
- Home visits – £30 per visit
- Full day including two visits – £500
- On call – additional £30 per hour
- Extra patients – £20 per patient
- Additional paperwork – charged at your hourly rate

For a long-term locum (i.e. a maternity locum), some GPs will negotiate to a slightly lower rate to give them the work security.

Remember that as a locum you won't be earning holiday pay, nor will you be earning study leave – keep this in mind when setting your rates. The average salaried GP will have 30 days' holiday a year, with an additional week of study leave on top of this. Thus, out of 52 weeks, you are working for 45 weeks. If you work, say, eight sessions at £500 per day, then you can work your yearly salary out as £90 000 per year. Obviously you will be paying your own General Medical Council registration and indemnity insurance, as well as for any continuing professional development you undertake. It has been said that a locum should earn approximately 30% more than a salaried GP to account for the uncertainty of being self-employed and for the loss of benefits you have of not having a contract to protect you.

Medeconomics magazine sometimes does surveys of locum earnings across the country. The last one was in May 2011 and this is available to view online – it is useful as a benchmark.

TERMS AND CONDITIONS

As with your rates, you too can be the author here. Once again, NASGP is a good place for guidance on this. Alternatively, there are plenty of freelance GPs who post their terms and conditions where you can access them online.

Things to include in your terms and conditions
- **Booking confirmation**: you can send a form for the practice to complete, sign and return to you confirming your appointment and their agreement to your terms and conditions prior to your arrival. Alternatively, you can email your terms and conditions and request a confirmation email in return, stating that they are in agreement.
- **Fees**: a breakdown of your fees (as stated earlier), including charges for additional extras (including extra patients, paperwork and visits).
- **Type of work**: state what you have agreed to – full (including appointments, telephone calls, administration, visits, on-call), surgery only (including associated administration time) or whatever else you have agreed to.
- **Dates and times**: be clear about the dates and the start and end times of your surgeries. It's embarrassing if and when this goes wrong!
- **Cancellation**: you can choose what you want to state here. You can charge a cancellation fee if your session is cancelled at short notice (i.e. 1 month before the locum date). Alternatively, you can invoice the surgery in full for your session or be generous and not charge at all.
- **Signing prescriptions**: your indemnity does not cover you to supervise other clinical staff, including those who may not be able to sign a script themselves (i.e. practice nurses). Therefore, you can refuse to sign these

prescriptions, or you can ask that the patient be added to your appointment list in order for you to review the case.

- **Parking/congestion charges**: if no parking is provided then you can include this in as an additional charge.
- **Surcharge for late payments**: you can expect to be paid within a specified amount of time (i.e. 28 days) once you have invoiced the practice; beyond that you can change a surcharge.

INVOICES AND ACCOUNTS

As a locum you will need to invoice each GP surgery for your time there. You need to include in the invoice the dates and rates of payment, and any additional payments incurred.

INVOICE

Dr New GP, MBChB, MRCGP   Tel: 0123456789
1 The Apartment, Central London, SW1   Email: newGP@nhs.net

To: Invoice No: 47
Practice Manager   Date: 15.01.12
The Local Medical Centre
1 The Road
London, SW1

Date	Session Details	Rate
02.01.12	Full day at The Local Medical Centre	£500
14.01.12	Half day at The Local Medical Centre, Including 2× visit @ £30 per visit	£310

Bank Details:	Subtotal	£810
The Bank and address.	VAT	£0
Account number and Sort code.	**Total**	**£810**

Please may I request this invoice be paid within 14 working days? I have enclosed a Pension Form A with the invoice. I would be grateful if you would complete this and return to my home address.

Keeping an accurate record of your work, creating your own invoices and keeping on top of this can be rather onerous and it's easy to fall behind with your administration. But fear not! There are plenty of companies out there that offer services for this, including:

- Locum Hub (www.locumhub.com)
- GP Advance (www.gpadvance.com)
- PennyPerfect (www.pennyperfect.co.uk).

YOUR PENSION

For each invoice you send to practices, include with it a Pension Form A. At the end of each month complete a Pension Form B and send this off with a cheque to the primary care trust. You will need to keep a record of these payments for your accountant. It is also important to complete these forms promptly, as some areas will not process late pension contributions. Additionally note that locum positions from a Primary Care Trust (PCT) point of view is a short-term role and if you are employed over a 3-month period, then they may question your role as a freelance GP. This may have implications for employer (PCT or the practice) contributions to your pension.

I have heard it asked before – would it be more lucrative for tax purposes to set yourself up as a limited company rather than being self-employed? However, you can only claim the NHS pension if you work for the NHS as an NHS employee or if self-employed, not as a private company. Therefore, this is a decision you will need to make with your financial advisor and accountant (given that the NHS pension is so good, my financial advisor advised me to stay with the NHS pension).

SUMMARY

Setting yourself up as a locum certainly has its advantages. If you choose to do this, the advice is:

- take the time to get in contact with local GP surgeries
- join local locum groups – good for networking, finding out what jobs are available, finding out the local rates, and for continuing professional development
- join NASGP
- be organised with your invoices, pension forms and finances
- make sure you book your holidays and days off in advance
- always have a 'savings bunker' to fall on in times of reduced work, illness or a very large tax bill.

Generally speaking, being a locum is a great experience, so give it a go.

REFERENCES

1 Balint, M. *The Doctor, His Patient and the Illness.* London: Routledge; 1956.
2 Tallis R. *Hippocratic Oaths: medicine and its discontents.* London: Atlantic Books; 2004.

C Salaried

Lindsay Moran, with input from Peter Davies

Pros	Cons
Guaranteed regular income	Less well paid
Maternity pay	Hard work, 'the dogsbody'
Continuity	Knowledge of one practice only
Get to know doctors and staff well	

There are a raft of good reasons to take up a job as a salaried doctor as a new GP. First, it gives you the opportunity to settle into a practice, get to know the staff, get to know the patients and start working towards contributing to your career development and that of the practice. You are protected from the practice business aspects at this stage, but if being a partner is your eventual goal then this is something you can work towards. It can be a great time to focus on improving your clinical care and focusing on your personal development plan to improve your skills as a doctor. Being a salaried GP is usually a comfortable option. Your time is guaranteed and this can be attractive if, for instance, you want to focus on your family.

As per the British Medical Association salaried contract, salaried GPs are employed for a defined number of hours per week (usually per session lasting 4 hours 10 minutes). You still need to be registered as a 'performer' with your local primary care organisation. The term 'salaried' can also refer to GP assistants, retainers and returners. Salaried GPs with freelance GPs come under the umbrella of sessional GPs.

IS BEING A SALARIED GP A GOOD ROUTE FOR A NEW GP TO TAKE?

The positives

Partnerships can be burdensome, especially for new GPs learning the ropes. Being a salaried GP takes away that burden, allowing the doctor to concentrate purely on their clinical work, with their free time to themselves – a definite bonus for those with family or other outside work commitments. For this reason, for younger GPs, and for older GPs nearing retirement who want more free time and a smaller workload, being salaried is a suitable first choice. Equally, for those needing more personal time to pursue a portfolio career, being salaried could allow for this.

Following the new GP contract in 2005, there has been an expansion in the number of salaried posts, meaning they are easier to come by than partnerships. That makes it easier to affiliate yourself with a practice you are likely to enjoy working at. For those as well who feel they are not in the position to cope with the responsibilities of being a partner and managing their own business, then this is a good option. Being resident at one practice allows for good continuity of practice and for you to build up your patient base. Being salaried gives a lot more flexibility than in partnership, allowing you to be more mobile about the country and also allowing flexibility with your hours, if this is what you need. The sessions can work around your lifestyle, whether that involves working around childcare and school hours or portfolio commitments.

The salaried contract can last for as long or as short a time as necessary for both parties. Leaving a practice requires only a short notice period. Your contract will, it is to be hoped, take into account paid continuing professional development (CPD) time, sick leave, study leave and maternity pay. Your income is not dependent on practice profits, and indemnity insurance is usually cheaper for salaried GPs. Banks also tend to be considerably happier to lend to a salaried GP than a freelance GP, if you are hoping to get a mortgage.

The negatives

The negatives include reduced commitment to the practice – you do 'just work there'. You do not have a say in how the practice runs or in how things get done. You have specific duties to your employer that may not benefit you much personally. A partner getting high Quality and Outcomes Framework scores will celebrate and will earn more. The salaried doctor may well regard the Quality and Outcomes Framework score with a certain indifference.

A salaried job may be working towards a partnership in the long term, but not always. After a few years in the job you may well be itching to move up into the partnership and the partners may want to keep you just where you are. Being salaried at the age of 30 may be OK, but by 35 you probably want to start developing your stake in the clinical and management processes of a practice. Staying salaried for too long may dissipate some of your early enthusiasm, and you may not get the chance to learn about practice development. Ultimately, most salaried jobs seem to last between 1 and 5 years and then the doctor moves on. Practices can view salaried GPs as lower status than freelance GPs.

As a GP partner, my (Peter's) observation on salaried jobs is that they are all right for a season of your career but they are unlikely to secure your lifelong commitment. Given that GP partnerships are about building care systems and practices over a long period of time, then the salaried option may not be your best long-term option.

The salaried option is a useful option at some stages of a career, but for those who want partnership it is worth knowing when to let it go. As a GP partner, if I have a salaried doctor whom I want to keep, I would want to turn him or her into a partner sooner rather than later.

Your pay may be lower than that of an equivalent partner post and you have no share in the profits. As you will be an employee, rather than self-employed, this has fewer tax allowances. If you have a specialist area of interest, such as minor surgery, it is to be hoped that your practice will support you in developing this, but this is not necessarily the case. Your opportunities for private work from the practice may be limited.

There is also the risk that the partners or employer can make you redundant.

INCOME

Being a salaried GP has benefits with regard to income (contrary to popular belief). You are guaranteed your income. This is unlike locuming or even in a partnership, where on a bad month the take-home pay could be less than the salaried GPs' pay.

It is often thought that salaried GPs earn significantly less than freelance GPs. Given that a salaried GP can negotiate their General Medical Council and indemnity payments, are covered for sick pay, holiday pay and maternity leave, and have a guaranteed monthly income, it works out that salaried GPs are not that badly off after all. Keeping up with the administration side of being a locum can take a significant chunk of time – this is something that the salaried GP is free from. Generally, a salaried GP earns less than the partners, but, equally, they have less business responsibility, so you would expect that to be the case. However, per hour, it is thought that salaried GPs actually earn more than some partners. When you consider the actual hours spent working for the take-home pay of salaried vs. partners, and when you take into account protected CPD time, the additional superannuation payments of partners and more recently the changes in taxation banding, you see rather surprisingly that salaried GPs may earn more per hour than their partner colleagues.[1]

Remember when comparing your PAYE salary with a partner's total income that the discrepancies may be explained by 'on-costs' (your employer's pension and National Insurance contributions), which may be about an extra 20% on top of your headline salary. Partners have to pay these themselves. Although the partners' 'profits' may look high, the drawings they can make on them may be surprisingly low when tax, National Insurance, pensions and other expenses have been paid.

At present, partner profits are being pushed down, and the salaried doctors may currently (November 2011) be in a better position than many partners, with more secure and possibly higher overall income. However, the balance of the earning potential of salaried vs. freelance vs. partnership earnings alters quite sharply when viewed over a 10- to 20-year time frame. This year's figures do not predict the future. Also, think about what you are building for the future.

CONTRACTS

You have a set contract and you are easily able to move practices if your personality does not suit the one you are currently at. The British Medical Association has a model salaried contract that practices are advised (but not necessarily obliged) to use. A job plan, stating duties of the salaried GP, should be agreed as part of the contract and this should not be an unlimited workload, as additional work is the responsibility of the partners.

CONTINUING PROFESSIONAL DEVELOPMENT

As part of your salaried contract you can expect to have CPD time written into this. This is generally easier to attend than when working as a locum. However, if you are working part-time to fulfil your CPD requirements for appraisal, a minimum of two sessions per week patient contact is recommended. As you are at one practice it is easier to follow up referrals and management plans for your experience.

REFERENCE

1 Slavin L. *Real Cost of Salaried GP vs Partner*. London: Ramsay Brown and Partners; 2009 November. Available at: www.ramsaybrown.co.uk/RealcostofsalariedGPvs Partner.htm (accessed 17 December 2011).

Chapter 7

Continuing professional development, appraisal and revalidation

Peter Davies, with input from Lindsay Moran

The important thing is never to stop questioning. Curiosity has its own reason for existing.

—Albert Einstein

In times of change learners inherit the earth while the learned are perfectly prepared for a world that no longer exists.

—Eric Hoffer

Nothing you will learn in the course of your studies will be of the slightest possible use to you in after life; save only this; that if you work hard and diligently you should be able to detect when a man is talking rot, and that, in my view, is the main, if not the sole purpose of education.

—Harold Macmillan, British prime minister, quoting one of his tutors in the classical languages and humanities

built-in, shock-proof, shit detector.

—Ernest Hemingway

INTRODUCTION AND OVERVIEW

This is a large and important chapter within this book.

In part it is positive, encouraging and, we hope, a spur to that lifelong curiosity that makes life more interesting and more fun. If the ideas in this chapter are approached positively you will have a more interesting career, enjoy meeting many different people, encounter many new ideas and end up treating your patients better. You will live in a lively intellectual and cultural milieu, and enjoy contributing to this and drawing resources from this.

In part it is a warning against complacency, and, we hope, a prophylactic against tedium, loss of interest, loss of engagement, withdrawal, isolation, burnout, depression and possible loss of concentration that can lead to poor performance.[1,2] As new GPs you probably have not been around long enough to see the end result of such processes, but at some stage you will observe these consequences taking a toll among some older GPs, many of whom are hoping to scrape by well enough to get to retirement safely.[3]

In part it is about two statutory processes, namely appraisal and revalidation.[4,5] Briefly, these processes are actually there to help you. As Matt Walsh, Colin Pollock and I put it in a *British Journal of General Practice* paper in 2011, *'The days of doctors being "good despite the system" should be going, and instead we should be able to say that doctors are good because of the system they work in.'*[6] They are the system attempts of the NHS and the General Medical Council (GMC) to help you with your ongoing professional development, either encouraging your existing efforts or reminding and encouraging you to do better. They are basically educational, and they are the first consciously created system to look at supporting doctors in an educational and to some extent pastoral manner.

Appraisal is not itself pastoral, but if problems are found earlier because of reflection during appraisal, then help and support can be mobilised before they become more major and cause damage either to the doctor's reputation or abilities or to any patients. One of the benefits of appraisal may be that it is allowing problems to be dealt with at an early stage when education and other supports are sufficient, and before the problem becomes worse and then the doctor has to be dragged into the disciplinary processes, or a partnership dispute. It is probably impossible to quantify this claim, but at the very least for doctors the appraisal process allows some time out for reflection and an opportunity to head problems off.

They are the first attempt by the NHS at any process of maintenance for the important asset that is medical professionals. In the old days (from 1948 to about 2002) it was largely assumed that professionals would maintain themselves, and that the 'odd failure or two' was acceptable attrition. It led to a phenomenon of battle-hardened cynical older doctors who were often in post as much for their ability at bluffing and toughing out the NHS as their clinical abilities.[7] Doctors who remained or became good doctors in such a system were good largely because of some inner personal resilience rather than because they worked in a system that made them good. Indeed, they were often good despite the system they worked within, and as a result often somewhat contemptuous of that system. Their retirement pieces and interviews often carry a 'Goodbye to all that' flavour about them.[8–10]

For new GPs, it is to be hoped you will not have that problem. You should in future find that you are working in a system within which your need for personal and professional development is actively acknowledged, although you will still have to negotiate to get exactly what you want when you want it.

We do in this chapter have to consider the clinical governance channels in play and how this affects your licence to practise medicine, and specifically general practice. The clinical governance system at your local primary care organisation describes the processes for dealing with complaints and other causes for concern. As a rule you need to be aware of such processes, and of how to largely avoid them.

Revalidation is a routine outcome of the processes of clinical professional development (as recorded via the appraisal system) and the local clinical governance processes. The GMC has long lamented that local clinical governance processes do not work as well as they could and so doctors who should be referred to them are not, and doctors whose cases should have been sorted locally end up being referred.

Revalidation is being introduced to give focus to local appraisal and clinical governance processes. The GMC[11] sees a four-layer model of professional regulation, starting with the doctor's own conscience, moving up to the peer pressure within the workplace, then to local regulation and finally, and only for severe issues, up to the national regulator – the GMC.

There are three possible outcomes to revalidation:

1. The responsible officer[12] has no option but to revalidate you if you have done your appraisals satisfactorily and there are no concerns from the performance management side. Most doctors should, and will, be in this group, and will know that they are in this group.

2. The responsible officer may defer your revalidation for a defined period in certain cases. These are likely to be cases where a doctor has been away for much of the preceding 5 years (e.g. for prolonged maternity leave or dealing with a health issue) and also where there is an ongoing complaint that needs resolution. In such cases the doctor's licence to practise remains completely intact, and it will be revalidated when the time comes.

3. The responsible officer may decide there is evidence of a failure to engage with the local clinical governance processes, including appraisal. This will

trigger concerns, although these concerns will probably have been triggered long before it gets anywhere near the revalidation decision.

The revalidation decision should be routine, humdrum and entirely expected. If there are surprises at that stage it would be seen as a failure of the local processes.

Revalidation is not intended to bring lots of GPs before the GMC's performance procedures. The GMC has no capacity to handle a rush of new cases. It is not meant to be onerous for any age of GP. Also, there is a service to keep running, and a developing shortage of GPs[13] and an increasing range of roles for us to deliver (as described in Chapter 4).

If there are concerns about a doctor's performance the local medical director should (and will) be acting on these as they arise, not once every 5 years when considering revalidation. In other words, if you are in trouble with performance issues you will know about it long before the revalidation decision.

So, the basic strategy for you as a new GP is to celebrate your new MRCGP certificate, keep on learning positively, keep on developing and avoid too many complaints.

Take part actively in the appraisal system. Always be looking to add to your value to patients and to potential employers by developing your skills and knowledge. It makes the job far more interesting, and it opens up new opportunities as you progress. Revalidation should just be routine for you.

However, if you decline to take part in continuing professional development, do not attend to your appraisals, demonstrate an unreflective attitude, and a general lack of insight, then you deservedly run a high risk of falling foul of local clinical governance processes and possible revalidation failure and/or referral to the GMC. You don't want that, do you?

As we move to consider these topics in more detail, the rest of this chapter is divided into the following topics:
a. Your licence to practise
b. Continuing professional development
c. Appraisal
d. Personal development plans
e. Revalidation
f. Clinical governance.

It shows how all of these are related to one another, and how crucial the roles of medical directors, appraisal leads and area educational tutors are currently – and how they will become even more important in time.

You will need to understand these topics as you work as a GP, and this chapter aims to provide a clear overview of what you will need to do in practice.

References and suggestions for further reading are given at the end of each section. Unavoidably, there is some overlap between the sections and their associated references.

REFERENCES

1 Ghodse H, Mann S, Johnson P, editors. *Doctors and their Health*. Sutton, Surrey: Reed Business Information; 2000.

2 Rowe L, Kidd M. *First Do No Harm: being a resilient doctor in the 21st century*. 1st ed. Maidenhead: McGraw-Hill Medical; 2009.

3 West L. *Doctors on the Edge: general practitioners, health and learning in the inner-city*. London: Free Association Books; 2001.

4 General Medical Council. *GP Framework for Appraisal and Revalidation*. London: GMC; 2011. Available at: www.gmc-uk.org/doctors/revalidation/revalidation_gmp_framework.asp (accessed 17 December 2011).

5 Royal College of General Practitioners. *Revalidation*. Available at: www.rcgp.org.uk/revalidation.aspx (accessed 17 December 2011).

6 Davies P, Walsh M, Pollock C. Performance management, appraisals, and revalidation: quantity analysis and quality control for UK GPs. *Br J Gen Pract*. 2011; **61**(589): 526–7.

7 Bennet G. *The Wound and the Doctor*. London: Secker & Warburg; 1987.

8 Riddell M. The *New Statesman* interview: Robert Winston. *New Statesman*. 2000 Jan 17. Available at: www.newstatesman.com/200001170011 (accessed 17 December 2011).

9 Dalrymple T. A doctor's farewell. *Spectator*. 2005 Jan 22. Available at: www.spectator.co.uk/spectator/thisweek/13125/a-doctors-farewell.thtml (accessed 17 December 2011).

10 Tallis R. *Hippocratic Oaths: medicine and its discontents*. London: Atlantic Press; 2005.

11 General Medical Council. *Memorandum by the General Medical Council (PS 92)*. London: 2011. Available at: www.publications.parliament.uk/pa/cm200809/cmselect/cmhealth/151/151we38.htm (accessed 26 April 2011).

12 National Archives. *The Medical Profession (Responsible Officers) Regulations 2010*. Available at: www.legislation.gov.uk/uksi/2010/2841/made (accessed 17 December 2011).

13 Mason R. Shortage of family doctors leaves health care in crisis. *Telegraph*. 2011 Dec 26. Available at: www.telegraph.co.uk/health/healthnews/8978509/Shortage-of-family-doctors-leaves-healthcare-in-crisis.html (accessed 17 December 2011).

A Your licence to practise

Peter Davies

As a new GP (or indeed as an established one, although some established GPs have not fully woken up to this reality and its implications yet) you need your licence to practise intact, and you need to be on a performer's list somewhere (or the equivalent in the devolved nations).

In the old days you got your licence to practise from the General Medical Council at full registration and then, provided you kept your nose clean, you and your employers could assume it was intact for your whole career.

These days you get your licence to practise, as a doctor generically and as a fully trained GP specifically. You also come under a local clinical governance process, and a local continuing professional development (CPD) and appraisal system. The local medical director is at the apex of this system, monitoring its outputs.

As a doctor your licence to practise is your most valuable asset, both for your professional pride and for your ability to earn a living from medicine. It can only be removed by the General Medical Council via its 'fitness to practise' procedures.[1,2] Like any asset it comes with a maintenance cost. You need to accept this maintenance cost; your practising privileges are granted on condition that you will pay heed to the need to maintain your licence. Alternatively, I should perhaps phrase it that it is a clear part of your role and duty as a doctor to show that you maintain yourself in a fit state of intellectual and professional relationship development so that you are able to do your job well.

You may well be (or be about to become) very busy seeing patients. You need to know you are doing this well, and in accordance with current standards and guidance. This means that at certain times you will need to break off from your busyness and see how well you are actually doing your business. This is in sharp contrast to the old days, where doctors were always busy – far too busy to interrupt this often unreflective business for any reason. Time out of surgery to do such reflective work should now be a routine part of normal clinical practice, and it should be counted as work or study leave, not as time off. Surgeries should be planning it into the working pattern of every doctor, and they should be keen to hear back the results from each individual doctor's learning and audits. In Peter Senge's phrase, surgeries need to be functioning as 'learning organisations'.[3] Currently some achieve this and some do not.

It is your responsibility as an individual doctor to pay the costs of keeping your licence intact willingly. If you are not willing to pay this cost then you deservedly run the risk that your licence will not be renewed. If professional status means anything it is a permanent and perennial concern about how well you do your job. Once you show signs of not caring about the quality of your work or not owning the results of your actions, you cease to really be a professional. You become a hollow mockery of a professional. You could, in Raymond Tallis's memorable phrase,[4] degenerate into a 'sessional functionary robotically following guidelines'.

To be professional is to be perennially self-critical, to always reflect on your actions and their outcomes, to always be learning, and to have a boundless curiosity that drives you to keep learning more. Once you are reduced to 'I only work here' and 'that's the way it is round here' or 'I'm always busy', you have given away or given up a part of your professional status and your stature is reducing.

In many ways a defining feature of professionalism is that your internal standards are so high that it becomes unnecessary and even counterproductive to supervise your work. In the old days of medicine this view was probably taken too far. Nowadays, your basic abilities will be accepted, but you may well be negotiating about where and to what purpose they need to be deployed.

Taking part in CPD and appraisal pays the cost of maintaining your licence to practise intact. The hope is that in the future the work you do personally as CPD will also help with input into area-wide service improvements as part of commissioning. If things work out well, then our individual and our collective efforts should become part of one whole.

REFERENCES

1 General Medical Council. *Good Medical Practice*. London: GMC; 2006. Available at: www.gmc-uk.org/static/documents/content/GMP_0910.pdf (accessed 17 December 2011).

2 Royal College for General Practitioners. *Good Medical Practice for General Practitioners*. London: RCGP; 2008. Available at: www.rcgp.org.uk/pdf/PDS_Good_Medical_Practice_for_GPs_July_2008.pdf (accessed 17 December 2011).

3 Senge P. *The Fifth Discipline: the art and practice of the learning organization*. London: Century Business; 1990.

4 Tallis R. *Hippocratic Oaths: medicine and its discontents*. London: Atlantic Press; 2005.

B Continuing professional development

Peter Davies, Hussain Gandhi and Lindsay Moran

So, as a newly qualified GP with a lovely new MRCGP certificate and an entry on the GMC specialist register, you are ready to be about your work. Complementing your practice, you have continuing professional development (CPD), which should be one of the joys of your medical career. It should also make your medical career more joyful. Appraisal and revalidation are basically about confirming that your CPD is happening, and that by reflection in action and reflection on action[1] you are actually learning from your experience. The alternative course – of repeating the same mistakes, not reflecting on them, and not learning from them – is the route to burnout, poor performance and a less enjoyable career for you.

CPD can be justified as a necessity. It is something that you have to do, to show that you are up to date, to get through appraisal and revalidation. However, this view presents it as a chore. Keep learning – it makes the whole job more interesting, coherent and fun. You chose to be a doctor, because whether because of the scientific or technical side or the patients or both, something about medicine brings you enjoyment and satisfaction. Your CPD should reflect this and should be something you find interesting, to be celebrated, and utilised. Your care to patients should be better as a result of your CPD.

In saying this I (Peter) am aware of how difficult it is to prove that CPD contributes to high standards of medical performance. On the other hand, I think the negative statement that doctors whose performance gives cause for concern often have CPD deficiencies is demonstrable. Would you rather be treated by a doctor who has made some effort to keep up to date through CPD or by a doctor who has ignored or avoided such processes?

Your CPD should be purposeful and it should show that you are meeting an educational need. This need may be personal or it may be shared with others (e.g. the practice); it may even be part of an area-wide project (e.g. for the local commissioning group). The better you can define your learning need or problem, the better you can tailor your plans to meet that educational need. Ultimately, you should be able to say why you are doing a particular learning activity, who the activity is for and who and what the activity will benefit.

The type of need to be met should also guide your technique for learning.

Some things go better to personal study and certain issues go better to discussion with colleagues.

Then you will have your personal learning style, which hopefully you will remember from your GP vocational training scheme days. Sometimes you are best to work with this, and sometimes the most learning comes from working with your opposite style or on a topic you are not much interested in – the effort forces you to find out why it matters and what you need to know about it. You can argue to soar with your strengths[2,3] or you can argue to learn to try and correct your current weaknesses. For most of us most of the time, I think the easiest way for CPD is to go with our preferred methods and styles, but be open to suggestions from others (e.g. an appraiser) that there may be other ways of doing things.

The better your CPD is, the better your learning will be. The more learned you are, the more effective you are, both in clinical practice and among colleagues. Dr Phil Hammond, comedian and GP, describes this as 'the mask of relaxed brilliance', but it takes a number of years to attain this; when you see someone who appears to have this facility, if you look closer you will find they have put much time and effort into obtaining it.[4,5]

There is a popular method of visualising the steps of learning in the form of a ladder. This 'ladder of competence' can be seen as moving from unconscious incompetence to conscious incompetence to conscious competence to unconscious competence and, finally, to a higher state where you become conscious about your unconscious competence. Basically, what this is describing is a journey from a state in which you are so ignorant that you do not even know there is a problem to one in which you become aware of the problem and want to do something about it. You then learn how to do it, but at this stage you have to think hard about each step you take. Think here of the difference between passing your driving test and how you drive now. Think of the difference between a new medical graduate and a seasoned registrar. They can both approach the same patients and problems, but the registrar will not have to think as hard as the new graduate will about what to do. Later on you reach unconscious competence – you just do the task and forget there was ever a time when you didn't know what a heart sounded like. When you have got to this level the danger is that you forget to appreciate how much you have learned to get there. Consciousness of your unconscious competence allows you to appreciate how far you have come, and how much you have learned. Humans have a tendency to discount what they have achieved, and to always want another problem or something new to tackle.[6] This is good, but every so often it is worth thinking consciously about how much you have already learned – don't just take it for granted. Teaching others is one great way to be reminded of this.

RECORDING AND REFLECTING ON YOUR CONTINUING PROFESSIONAL DEVELOPMENT

It is not enough just to do your CPD and to record it. It is also necessary to reflect on it. By reflection here we mean something that might read as follows:

> I discovered that we had a group of patients with untreated high lipid levels in our practice (*a clinical need*). I read the available guidance and a recent review article about this topic (*information-gathering stage*). I also spoke with the local lipid specialist (*you learn a lot from conversations*). Following on from this I discussed the issue with my colleagues (*teamwork and reflection in action*). We agreed to make a change in our practice so that if we see anyone in this patient group we will now treat them actively, and follow them up more intensely. We ran an audit after this and the numbers going undertreated have now reduced from y to x.

In an instance like this you have engaged purposeful CPD that is not only relevant to the individual doctor but also relevant to the practice and what it does. It meets a need for a group of patients. Ideally, CPD can be shown to meet an educational need and to have within it the possibility of better patient care.

By looking at the initial problem definition and the learning points and action points that arise as a result of the CPD time spent on the problem, reflection can be shown. Fundamentally, CPD is learning undertaken for a purpose, and not just for personal interest or amusement.

For appraisal and revalidation purposes appraisers are hoping to see CPD become more focused and purposeful. We want to see a move away from a folder of certificates of various meetings attended because they were available, at a nice venue, with nice food laid on. We are also keen to see personal activity and reflection and not doctors hiding in the wake of their other colleagues.

Personal reading of, for example, the *BMJ* each month can count as CPD. However, such activity is useful scanning rather than great CPD. As an appraiser, if you told me you searched the *BMJ* and other relevant journals looking for information about a specific topic that had come up in practice then I would see that as much more focused and purposeful. Reading is a good way for many of us to learn and it is classed as structured or unstructured. Structured reading is reading to find out information about a specific problem. Unstructured reading is general scanning of the medical journals each week or month. It is allowable for CPD but only to a maximum of 10 credits per year.

CPD can be done for many reasons and to meet many needs. For new GPs the important thing is to keep your curiosity intact, and always be looking to improve your knowledge and skills. As a new GP many topics may still be new to you. And that includes many bits of clinical practice and then probably all the management side of your job. It is to be hoped that this book will speed up your acquisition of some of these skills. As a new GP you will have no shortage of CPD topics to choose from. One of the main jobs of an appraiser is to help you sort out your list of priorities, and to turn them into manageable chunks that can be measured and completed.

The following list shows some of the many activities that can be counted as CPD:
- private study
- reading
- educational modules
- educational courses
- professional meetings with colleagues
- time spent on clinical audit and significant event audit
- practice team learning and development (not routine business) meetings
- conferences
- time spent on teaching and training
- time spent on area-wide development activities (e.g. as part of commissioning)
- academic activity is allowable (e.g. research and writing it up).

LEARNING CREDITS

CPD activity is measured by means of learning credits.[7,8] The aim is to have a minimum of 50 credits per year and 250 credits per 5-year revalidation cycle. You can do some trading between years over the 5-year revalidation cycle to reach the 250 total. However, for most doctors it is sensible to aim to gather learning credits steadily over the years.

Basically, one credit is awarded for **1 hour of CPD** activity that is **recorded**, with **documented reflection in place**. You need to show why you did that particular piece of CPD activity, what educational need it met, what you learned from it and what action you will take as a result. The days of CPD being an activity that merely involves attending meetings have gone.

If a learning activity can be shown to have had an impact beyond itself and the individual doctor, the learning credit claim can be doubled. Impact here would be in terms of improved patient care, a new system within a practice, or a major piece of leadership that affects many people. Almost all GP educational activity qualifies for double impact under this criterion. The impact needs to be demonstrable in some way.

Learning credits are verified each year by your appraiser.

On a practical note, it is worth saying that although many of us do way more CPD than 1 hour per week, we do not all record it properly or reflect on it fully.

In future, for CPD and for appraisal and revalidation, it will pay GPs to record properly between 50 and 100 credits' worth of CPD. Anything less than 50 credits is not enough, especially if the appraiser challenges any items on your list. Anything over 100 credits is too much for your appraiser to read, and, indeed, may not be well recorded or reflected on.

RECORDING CONTINUING PROFESSIONAL DEVELOPMENT

Newly qualified GPs will probably be more adept at keeping their CPD record up to date than most of their older colleagues. They are likely to be more au fait with the ePortfolio[8] or similar systems[9] than the more weathered GPs. Like the ePortfolio, keeping up to date with your record of CPD events as you go along is generally better than a mad last-minute panic at the end, trying to remember everything you've been up to for the last year. Some good tips are simply to regularly log in to wherever you store your information and update it, to keep a little diary with you and write something for each event you attend, or, even better, write it all up on your smartphone notes when you are at the event (many GPs do this now).

Keeping a good record of your CPD will lead nicely into your appraisal. There are various toolkits to record your CPD, in various stages of development, and there are pros and cons to them all (not least of all that some you need to pay for!). The good toolkits should allow you to record the basic CPD details: date, time spent, meeting title, credits claimed. However, they should go on to ask you the reflective questions:
- Why did you choose to do this piece of CPD?
- What was your learning need here?
- What did you learn about the topic?
- What actions are you now going to take?

In other words, they make it easy for you to reflect and record your reflection on your learning processes and on what you are taking out from your CPD activity. They make it easier for you to reflect than not, and from the processes of reflection and subsequent action emerges the true value of CPD.

The RCGP toolkit[8] is an ongoing work, and similar in architecture to the ePortfolio you will know from your GP training days. As a system it is getting better, but it still feels clunky and slow. It has certain good points (particularly its CPD logging) and the number of prompts it gives you to record reflections and learning points. All personal development plan goals have to be suggested by the appraisee ahead of the appraisal interview (I think this is a strength of the system, provided appraisees are up to speed on this). Its weaknesses are its slowness and its pedantry, and sometimes the processes of logging in and signing off are difficult.

The old NHS Appraisals website has a new product,[9] and this may be a good future option. It charges a subscription and also quite a high charge to the primary care trust for the administrator function. You need to know locally which appraisal toolkits your primary care trust supports.

The need for toolkits for appraisal and revalidation is there, but which product will be the best one to use is currently (April 2012) far from clear. Other options are provided by various institutions, including the new BMJ e-portfolio, which has a focus on multidisciplinary learning, and the excellent GPtools.[10] This is a free resource created by a GP, with a clean interface and ease of use. I (Hussain), highly recommend using this site, especially if you do not wish to pay for an ePortfolio. Additionally both of these ePortfolios can be easily exported as PDFs for printing, if your primary care trust does not support either of these two options.

For the time being, some doctors have returned to paper in folders, using the appraisal requirements as a guide. This may make sense for now (2011–13), but in the long run it is a backward step.

METHODS OF CONTINUING PROFESSIONAL DEVELOPMENT

Courses

There are many courses that run up and down the country catering to a host of CPD needs. These can target specific clinical or managerial areas, or they can be update courses for the busy clinician. Ideally these courses will be chosen by you strategically to meet an expressed learning need, e.g. 'I went on this course to learn how to initiate insulin prescribing safely and sensibly from my surgery. Since going on it I now do . . .'

In response to the need for additional support to newly qualified GPs, the RCGP holds courses aimed specifically at their First5® initiative.[11]

Reading

For many, reading on a topic can provide a quick and efficient way to learn about it.

This can be from recognised journals (e.g. *BMJ, Lancet, British Journal of General Practice, InnovAiT* and so forth) or from books. However, with the internet available in most of our consulting rooms, looking at other alternatives may be useful. One way is to create a personal web magazine using a news feed aggregator that brings information from various resources such as Flipboard, *Pulse* or Google Reader. Using combined RSS (really simple syndication) feeds, which are regularly updated news feeds from a provider such as *GP* online, BMJ, BBC Health and so forth, can allow you to create your own tailored journal to read. When combined with an offline reader (i.e. Instapaper or Read It Later), they can make a simple, portable way of bringing information on various topics to your fingertips.

Remember the difference between unstructured browsing and purposeful literature searching for specific learning needs.

E-learning

If you wish to learn something more specific, e-learning modules can offer more targeted learning, combined with assessments that normally give credits based on the time spent working through the module. There are many providers of these, including eGP (the RCGP online learning environment, www.e-GP.org), 'doctors.net' (www.doctors.net.uk/), BMJ online modules (http://learning.bmj.com/learning/home.html) and Pri-Med Coffee Break Learning (www.pri-medupdates.co.uk/ecme/video). These can offer a wealth of evidence-based resources, and are often well referenced, with the recent links and references easily accessible.

In addition, there are the clinical updates that are online, like the very successful RCGP Essential Knowledge Update programme or more facilitated/blended learning courses like the Medical Update or institution-based courses (i.e. MSc/PG Cert courses).

There are a variety of web-based clinical resources at your disposal that can be used both for CPD information and for clinical information finding. Well-known sites include GPnotebook (www.gpnotebook.co.uk), Clinical Knowledge Summaries (www.cks.nhs.uk) and Patient.co.uk. However, if you are searching for a good portal for these resources and other options, you can try reference websites such as eGP Learning (www.egplearning.co.uk).

Capturing information from colleagues

Some reading this chapter will think this is purely around the technology, but some of the most impactful learning we have is when we hear from colleagues or specialists in person. Capturing information from colleagues has always been a little trickier. For these instances, while pen and paper with the odd voice recorder may be useful, I recommend trying various notepad applications. Such examples of Evernote, or Springpad, can allow you to write or even dictate into a notepad from most mobile or internet-connected devices. This information is then stored securely online, and can even have photos or video footage added. Using this method can then easily lead into the appropriate portfolio of your choice. This method of recording can also be very effective when attending conferences or clinical/practice meetings.

New media

New media has also lead to an explosion of methods of CPD learning. Podcasts (audio tutorials) and vodcasts (video and audio tutorials) or webinars (live online tutorials) are fast becoming a method of supporting individual learning needs.

Again, there is a wealth of providers including the NHS, Podmedics and the likes of various clinical skills tutorials on YouTube.

Social networking

But why limit yourself? Social networking has broken down the limits of meeting face to face, with pioneering projects such as Twitter Journal Club (@twitjournal club, #twitjc), which provides the opportunity to take part in an online medical journal club with a variety of colleagues over the world. This has lead to an expanding model such as the regular running #gasclass for anaesthetic doctors. Following the relevant hashtag on Twitter means participation, with concise engagement, and extractable dialogue for enhanced CPD reflections.

Our RCGP chair Dr Clare Gerada (@clarercgp) is a prolific tweeter, as are many other UK GPs (including our own Hussain Gandhi – @drgandalf52 and Lindsay Moran – @lindsmoran). RCGP First5® also has its own following (@rcgpfirst5) – I would recommend you follow this, as well as joining their Facebook group. The Yorkshire First5® group is kept in contact via social networking. However, if you prefer the face-to-face option, make sure to seek out your local CPD group.

The key point amidst all these technical innovations is to remember that you need to know what you need to learn, and why you are doing it. Once you know this you can then choose the method to meet the need.

CONTINUING PROFESSIONAL DEVELOPMENT GROUPS

Working as a GP can at times be isolating, so getting involved with a CPD group may be good for your personal development, your networking and for sharing ideas among colleagues. These groups have existed in a number of guises all over the country, brandishing names from 'young GPs' groups' (which makes it harder to adhere to the name as time passes and more grey hairs appear) to 'local sessional groups'. Often friends and colleagues leaving the vocational training scheme start groups and continue to meet up. Different parts of the country have different set-ups with their CPD groups, with some groups open to new members and some closed. If you're new to an area or simply want to join an established group then your three best sources of information for local groups are:

1. your First5® representative at the local RCGP faculty (www.rcgp.org.uk/college_locations/faculties.aspx)
2. the National Association of Sessional GPs – the website lists the national groups available to join, although this list is by no means complete (www.nasgp.org.uk/)
3. word of mouth via other GPs.

It is often advisable to be part of a CPD group. As well as educational support they are also good for emotional support. Many doctors who have serious complaints brought against them are often found to be locally isolated. However, as the fell-walker Alfred Wainwright once pointed out, 'I am never lonelier than when in a crowd'. You can be in a group of colleagues and still be very isolated.

When you attend your group, you need to record what it is you have discussed. It is a good idea to keep a signed register as record of attendance. The RCGP has published a guide for recording your CPD sessions and it is available from the First5® and revalidation sections of their website.

In addition to this guide, you may wish to generate learning needs from each session and an agenda for your next session.

Lindsay

I am lucky to be part of two CPD groups in Leeds. The first is a large sessional GPs' group that is open to all and attended by a range of sessional GPs across the area. I am generally the youngest at these sessions. I have learned a great deal clinically from the more experienced GPs, but more so I have taken away a huge amount of practical advice with regard to working as a locum GP in terms of rates, terms and conditions and so forth.

My second group is a small closed group made up of a few vocational training scheme friends. We meet each month at a different person's house, order pizza, then take it in turns to do presentations on whatever we feel is relevant. We use the aforementioned pro forma at each session and we generate an agenda for the next session based on queries that have come up in the session (i.e. how to investigate and treat vitamin D deficiency, consideration of the use of HbA1c in the diagnosis of diabetes, new National Institute for Health and Clinical Excellence guidelines and so forth). We also discuss significant events. Using Google Sites, we have made a purpose-built website to record each session, such that is accessible to all and we can upload all documents and presentations.

Hussain

I am fortunate to be part of several groups. I participate in similar groups to Lindsay, but one is based in the Bradford and Airedale region, which is smaller than the Leeds group but which offers a more personal approach (meetings are based at members' houses every 6 weeks). I engage with the revalidation group within the Academic Unit of Primary Care in Leeds where I work, and the practice-based educational learning. I also find benefit from attending locally provided educational events, by local GPs such as a successful update course, hot topics and even secondary care teaching at grand rounds.

CONCLUSION

We hope this chapter has shown you what CPD is about and some of the ways in which it done. Rather than just attending a random spectrum of meetings or doing a random selection of modules, the key point is to have a purpose to your CPD activities.

REFERENCES

1 Schon D. *The Reflective Practitioner: how professionals think in action.* New ed. Avebury: Ashgate Publishing; 1991.
2 Clifton DO, Nelson P. *Soar with Your Strengths: a simple yet revolutionary philosophy of business and management.* New York: Dell Publishing; 1996.
3 Buckingham M, Clifton DO. *Now, Discover Your Strengths: how to develop your talents and those of the people you manage.* London: Pocket Books; 2005.
4 Colvin G. *Talent is Overrated: what* really *separates world-class performers from everybody else.* London: Nicholas Brealey Publishing; 2008.
5 Syed M. *Bounce: the myth of talent and the power of practice.* London: Fourth Estate; 2011.
6 Schulz K. *Being Wrong: adventures in the margin of error.* London: Portobello Books; 2010.
7 Royal College of General Practitioners. *Guide to the Credit-Based System for CPD.* Version 2.0. London: RCGP; 2010. Available at: www.rcgp.org.uk/PDF/Credit-Based%20System%20for%20CPD_2nd%20version_110110.pdf (accessed 3 April 2012).
8 Royal College of General Practitioners. *Revalidation ePortfolio* [online tool]. Available at: https://gpeportfolio.rcgp.org.uk (accessed 3 April 2012).
9 https://appraisals.clarity.co.uk
10 www.gptools.org
11 www.rcgp.org.uk/new_professionals/first5.aspx

C Appraisal

Peter Davies, with input from Lindsay Moran

Your appraisal each year is basically a check that the continuing professional development (CPD) processes as already described are happening. They do not all have to happen each year. However, over the 5-year revalidation cycle, each area should be covered at least once.

At its best, appraisal is a formative developmental process in which the appraisee can reflect and learn from their experience with the help of an experienced and well-trained colleague. The process is supportive, helpful and friendly, and is basically a purposeful meeting of colleagues. It is confidential, with agreed developmental outcomes for the following year. Think of it as a journey with a pit stop to see whether you are on the right path or not.

It is a once-a-year event, and although a case could be made in some instances to extend it into mentoring or coaching, there is no current plan or provision for this to happen. The process remains a useful annual event at which a doctor can review their professional progress and plan what their CPD topics and processes need to be over the coming year. **For all that the appraisal interview is an annual event, it is worth treating the CPD and other preparation for the interview as an ongoing process throughout the year.**

KEY POINTS ABOUT APPRAISAL
- Own your appraisal – this is an opportunity for you.
- It's a continuous process and not just an interview once a year.
- Keep it personal – it's about you, not them.
- A small amount of personally relevant material with reflection, learning points and action points is what the appraisers want to see.
- Revalidation is a minor event, but one that reflects and confirms that important underlying professional processes are in place.
- The system and those of us running it want you to perform well and to help you maintain that high standard.
- All the appraisal and CPD activity you do is ultimately about improving the service you can provide to patients.

There are some specific requirements for appraisal and we describe these shortly, along with some suggested smart strategies for making it easy to gather the required information.

For those of you who are very busy, this summary from the *Calderdale Appraisal Guide 2012–13* points out the basics quickly.

- Appraisal is a professional obligation under performers list regulations. Not taking part risks your status on that list and thereby your licence to practise.
- More positively, it is an opportunity to reflect on your work, and a system that will help you to do it better in the future, increasing your satisfaction and enjoyment, and it is to your patient's benefit.
- Revalidation is a simple decision: if you keep your CPD and appraisals up to date and avoid performance management issues, the responsible officer, whoever he or she is, has to revalidate you.
- The appraisal evidence headings[1,2] and the questions being asked of you are now:
  - Continuing professional development – What am I doing to keep up to date and to improve?
  - Clinical audit (performance measurement) – What are my current standards of practice like?
  - Significant event audit (SEA) – What do I do about unusual events?
  - Multi-source feedback (MSF) – How do I come across to my colleagues?
  - Patient feedback (PF) – How do I come across to my patients?
  - Response to complaints and concerns – How have I handled concerns about my work?
- The emphasis throughout is on demonstrating reflection and learning, and actions taken in response to identified problems.
- The appraiser's job is to help you get that process of reflection right, and to focus it into useful educational activities that meet your educational needs.
- The appraisal process is about the individual doctor.
- The hope is that, in the future, the work you do as CPD will also help with input into area-wide service improvements as part of commissioning. If things work out well then our individual and our collective efforts should become part of one whole.

WHAT YOU NEED TO DO TO PREPARE FOR THE APPRAISAL INTERVIEW

Your CPD is an ongoing process. You need to get a system in place for recording your CPD and your reflections upon it. You do not want to be gathering a large amount of material together in a folder less than 1 week before the appraisal. The material wants to be personal to you, and specific to your educational needs and the aforementioned summarised points. It does not want to be the whole practice complaints, clinical audit and SEA file – just those selected bits from the whole practice file that you were personally involved with. The fact your event has been reviewed by the practice is good – it is evidence of shared learning and teamwork. However, remember appraisal is about reviewing you and your work, not the whole practice.

There is a significant debate among appraisers as to how far you can isolate the individual doctor and their evidence, outcomes and results from their practice. To a large extent we all achieve through teamwork. Indeed, it is likely that a poorer doctor among better colleagues will perform better overall than a better doctor among poorer colleagues. Whatever the outcome of this debate, the current advice to appraisees is that, as far as you can, present a selected folder of information that is personally relevant to you, not a profile of your whole practice.

It is worth thinking before your appraisal interview about what you have done so far, and what areas you need to cover next year. Having a list of topics or a suggested personal development plan is very helpful to the appraiser.

It is very important that you look over last year's form 4 and PDP before your appraisal interview and present them as part of your appraisal evidence. In particular consider whether you have met last year's PDP goals and expect to be asked about them.

You need to get your evidence to your appraiser at least 2 weeks before your appraisal.

THE APPRAISAL PAPERWORK

As with all processes, there is associated paperwork with the appraisal. We have classically had forms 1–5.

- Form 1 is basic demographic details (name, address, General Medical Council number and so forth).
- Form 2 is basic workplace information (your surgery address, what you do, additional activities and so forth). It needs to include a full description of your work in all its aspects, and not just your work in your main surgery, such as teaching, research, GPwSI (GP with a special interest) and so forth.
- Form 3 is the appraisee's reflective commentary on their work over the last year. It is written under the headings of 'Good clinical care', 'Keeping up to date', 'Relationships with patients', 'Relationships with colleagues', 'Management (outside the practice)', 'Teaching and training', 'Research', 'Probity and health'.
- Form 4 is the appraiser's summary of the appraisal discussion with specific references to evidence seen in Form 3, issues arising, learning needs identified, and items to take forward as part of the personal development plan. It is an important document; it will be checked for quality and will often be used by the medical director if any concerns emerge about a doctor. A Form 4 is as notable for what goes unsaid, as what is said.

- Form 5 is for information that is entirely private between appraise and appraiser. This form is rarely used, as such information tends not to get written down at all.

Completing the forms

OK, so how do you set about answering all the questions in the forms to demonstrate you are a good, well-rounded, up-to-date doctor for your appraisal? The answer is with evidence, and this evidence should be personal to you. A small amount of personally relevant information is much more useful than the whole practice's SEA, clinical audit and complaints file. Appraisal is about you as an individual doctor.

Given that the bulk of the appraisal will focus on Form 3 or its later equivalents, we shall concentrate on this.

Now, there was a good side to the Form 3 headings: they allowed the appraisee to reflect widely on their work. Some doctors did this very well, whereas others floundered, guessing what was needed under each heading with varying success. There was an equally bad side to them in that they allowed the appraisee to reflect widely, to waffle, and to little purpose, in an evidence-free way. When you write you give away a lot of evidence about yourself and your character. In appraisal you are supposed to document specific points that show how well or otherwise your medical practice is going.

The new toolkits are moving much more towards specific information recording. This is good in that it forces the appraisee to present evidence. It is poor in that it stops the wider reflections that are sometimes insightful. There is a balance to be struck between including specific evidence to show what you are saying and allowing more general overall commentary about the whole of your work. As an example, an audit of management of high cholesterol will be interesting, but it is clearly only a part of a doctor's work and so it would leave much unsaid about that larger whole. Aim to demonstrate not only what you have learned over the last year but also how your practice has improved.

The new GMC headings clump the evidence into four larger domains.[1,2]

Domain 1: Knowledge, skills and performance
attribute 1.1, professional performances
attribute 1.2, knowledge and experience
attribute 1.3, records

Domain 2: Safety and quality
attribute 2.1, patient protection and improved care
attribute 2.2, risk management
attribute 2.3, own health

Domain 3: Communication, partnership and teamwork
attribute 3.1, communications
attribute 3.2, colleagues and delegation
attribute 3.3, patient partnerships

Domain 4: Maintaining trust
attribute 4.1, respect for patients
attribute 4.2, fairness
attribute 4.3, honesty/integrity

These new headings do not now cover the whole of many GPs' work, and sections such as education and teaching, management outside the practice and research largely disappear. Some of this activity is assessed and appraised elsewhere and some just seems to vanish off the radar.

There are certain specific areas that it is necessary based on General Medical Council guidance[1,2] to cover via CPD and the appraisal system:

Continuing professional development (Do I keep up to date?)
Showing you are up to date is easily demonstrated with a well-maintained CPD log. Your CPD log should show what you have done, and it should contain some reflection and learning and action points from your learning activity. We all learn in different styles, but the appraiser is looking for evidence of ongoing learning, in a style that works for you. Your CPD should be specifically relevant to your identified learning needs. It is advisable to record your CPD regularly, with ongoing reflection, and notes of learning and action points identified. Ideally, the CPD log is maintained electronically and the whole reflected on at least annually at the appraisal.

Quality improvement activity
This is personal to you as far as possible. It needs to be an accurate recording of team and individual reflection. We are not planning to say much about the mechanics of clinical audit or SEA here. It is to be hoped that you already know this from your training; if not, then the references at the end should help you.

Clinical audit (Is my clinical care good enough?)
Now, you cannot audit every area of your practice, but you can audit some areas. Evidence that you are looking at what you are doing, comparing it with recommended standards such as National Institute for Health and Clinical Excellence guidance, and acting to remedy any gaps found is reassuring.

Significant event audit (Do I respond to signals of the unusual?)

The appraiser is likely to ask you what you do when something unusual crosses your path. Who or what do you turn to? What do you do about it? How do you find out if the unusual is an isolated incident or an area-wide problem?

Doing an SEA is fun and it can be on almost anything. If I (Peter) am looking for significant events, I reckon I could find about 10 incidents worth reviewing in any week in practice. The revalidation requirement is 10 in 5 years. Some of my colleagues probably think I have an eventful life, but actually the doctor who is willing to discuss and learn from significant events is the one who is stronger. It may well be that the doctors and the practices that have more SEAs are the ones more tuned in to the risks and events in their practice, and actually practising a lot more safely than doctors and practices with seemingly fewer events.[3,4]

SEA is a great technique that uses as a resource for learning the specific examples and stories that are so much a feature of GP life. The problem with SEA is that no one is sure what the threshold for 'significant' is, and therefore at what level it is worth bringing an event to the larger practice. The National Patient Safety Agency has produced useful guidance on this process.[5] Worries about risks to reputation, risks of legal disclosure, not wanting to rock the boat and so on all lead to doctors hiding away examples that people could learn from in their private experience. Too much in medicine is shrugged away privately as 'just the way it happens round here'. The joy of good colleagues is that you form a learning organisation,[6] and you learn from one another. Sitting in judgemental, fearful, self-censored silence from one another is not the sign of a dynamic learning organisation.

EVIDENCE OF REFLECTION ON HOW YOU COME ACROSS TO OTHERS

The processes for this Multiple Source Feedback (MSF) and Patient Source Feedback (PSF) are not yet fully developed. They are potentially very useful tools giving us much information about how we come across to others. And yet they are being introduced, and few doctors are trained in giving MSF well and fewer are well trained in interpreting it. It is not clear who should own the feedback evidence, or whether it should be edited before it is given to the appraisee. There are concerns about its accuracy, ranging from 'sharp and deadly' to 'sharp and supportive' to 'risks becoming a bit bland and generic'.

As appraisers we are not fully sure how we will manage these processes well enough, to get full value out of them. New GPs are at an advantage, having gone through similar feedback processes during their training.

The basic point here is that, as doctors, we need some idea about how we are perceived by others. We then need to know if our perceptions of ourselves match those of patients and colleagues, and then to see if we can explain either good matches or significant mismatches. As in so much adult education, and good professional practice, the emphasis here is on reflection leading to insight, learning and improvement.

Marshall Goldsmith has written a good book on MSF[7] and it has the great title of *What Got You Here Won't Get You There*. Goldsmith's key point is that most of us have got to where we are partially because of who we are and our great knowledge and talents and partially because other people have been kind enough to ignore or work around our ignorance, foibles and unpleasant idiosyncrasies. Perhaps with PSF and MSF we will be able to develop our good points further and in turn knock some of the rough edges off our bad points. Goldsmith mainly works with senior managers at the level just below senior directors, and those who may be the next people to come through as senior directors. At the lower levels, and hidden within an organisation, these people's idiosyncrasies may be tolerable, but once they are in an exposed position as a chief executive officer or similar their foibles could become major issues that could threaten the viability of their organisations. In our work as GPs we are moving ever more into leadership roles such as commissioning, so getting used to PF and MSF could be a useful step in every GP's development.

The approved tools for PSF by PSQ (the Patient Satisfaction Questionnaire) and MSF are now available on the RCGP website.[2]

For revalidation the requirement at present is to take part in the MSF and PSQ. There are no specific scores or thresholds. However if the feedback is unfavourable or critical and raises issues about a doctor's performance then it may become a route by which a concern about performance could arise.

If, when giving, feedback you are at the level of saying severely critical things about a colleague's performance such as 'I do not think he or she can make even the most basic diagnosis' then you are really at the level of having a performance concern about that colleague, and you should then stop the MSF, and take advice from your Medical Defence Organisation and the Medical Director about how to proceed. There is new GMC guidance on this topic (March 2012). The link is www.gmc-uk.org/Raising_and_acting_on_concerns_about_patient_safety_FINAL.pdf_47223556.pdf.

On the whole the best advice about giving MSF seems to be to keep the feedback about behavioural issues, rather than identity or character issues. Suggestions for improvement may be accepted and implemented. The advice is to give feedback in such a way that you help your colleague to improve. Direct feedback about each other's character flaws is unlikely to help any of us, and indeed there is concern at senior levels that such direct critical feedback could actually be damaging to the person receiving it, or giving it. Please use MSF to help colleagues improve.

EVIDENCE OF RESPONSE TO CONCERNS: REFLECTION ON COMPLAINTS AND COMPLIMENTS

The key issue here is to show that you are learning something from complaints and compliments. Although complaints are unpleasant at first, with the passage of time and with further reflection a certain amount of learning can come from them.

For appraisal and revalidation purposes the aim is to show that complaints are noted, responded to professionally and that something is learned from them – even if that is simply how to avoid the particular issue in future.

Some medical directors write to doctors on their performers list and ask for specific items or questions to be reviewed in an educational way at appraisal. Such suggestions go to the appraisee directly, and the appraisee then has an option whether to include the items or not among his or her evidence for appraisal. The medical director's suggestions may include reviewing a complaint or some outlying figures (e.g. on prescribing). Often, the medical director will have no specific items to suggest; in this case the letter will simply confirm that no specific concerns are present.

The key with events that may raise concerns such as complaints, or negligence actions, is to realise that they are not bad in themselves. Identifying outlying performance is also an opportunity at an early stage to prevent future complaints and negligence. Running such events through the CPD and appraisal channels allows the doctor to show that they are learning from experience, and are handling such events sensibly – both in terms of providing professional and accurate responses to patients at risk and in terms of looking after themselves through what can be upsetting experiences for the doctor. Your appraiser can often help you make better sense of such events, and such support is often welcomed. Your appraiser may help put you in touch with people or resources that can help you.

All of us will receive some complaints during our career. If we handle these concerns well we come across as intelligent, reflective doctors who learn as we go on. We will not raise concerns about our performance; indeed, the act of showing that we have reflected on adverse outcomes and taken appropriate remedial actions to reduce future risk to patients shows us demonstrating good medical practice in action.

If we handle these concerns poorly (e.g. by denying such events, or by learning nothing from them), we potentially show ourselves to be arrogant, ignorant and unreflective doctors. If such behaviour reaches the point of 'lack of insight' then medical directors will grow concerned and rightly consider investigating your performance further. As a sensible doctor, surely you don't want to raise their concerns about you, do you?

All the learning activities here are not ends in themselves. For each of them the appraiser is keen to see evidence of reflection, lessons learned, and changes made in practice. The aim here is continuous quality improvement, and if you identify a problem and do nothing about it then nothing is really learned either by the individual doctor or the system. Considering your actions in your clinical activity and how you have improved can show this well, as can keeping a list of PUNs and DENs (patients' unmet needs and doctors' educational needs)[8] to show your reflection on your knowledge base.

The key driver of learning at appraisal is the concept from Donald Schon of 'reflection in action'.[9] The idea here is that professionals do an activity, gather feedback and then work out if they are doing well or could do it better. They then adjust their performance on the next cycle. What appraisal is looking for is evidence of reflective practice – that you have considered if you may be mistaken, if you have learned from experiences, events, colleagues and patients. The assumption here is that a reflective doctor who is learning continuously is probably a good one.

The alternative of the unreflective practitioner, one who cannot see his or her mistakes and so keeps repeating them without insight, is a risky doctor. Any medical director will tell you that an unreflective doctor is one of the warning signs that may alert them to critically review, and perhaps investigate, that doctor's performance.

For appraisers, the main worry is if there is no presentation of data or information.

HELP! IT'S MY FIRST APPRAISAL AS A QUALIFIED GP

Relax. The first appraisal after MRCGP is a slightly odd one. You have just been validated by a formal exam. We know you are up to date – it is only a year (at most) from when you passed the MRCGP. Your appraiser knows you are a new GP and therefore that you will not have much of a portfolio to show just yet, unless you recycle all your registrar work – this work will not interest your appraiser much, and it has already been assessed. You may well not be fully settled in a practice, and you are probably struggling with your first steps in the profession.

Apart from anything else, appraisal is a great opportunity to meet and learn from colleagues. As an appraiser I often learn more from the person I am appraising and their practice than what I contribute. Some of my most useful appraisals have been ones I have done for new GPs.

What appraisals offer is the chance for you to meet with an experienced senior colleague who usually has some knowledge of the local area and the practice you are in. He or she will find out about the exact working situation you are currently in. Once your situation is defined then practical steps such as additional learning can be considered, and a personal development plan developed that, it is to be hoped, helps you address what you need to find out about.

The first appraisal is often as much teaching as appraising, and about helping young colleagues to understand appraisal and what they need to get together for the year after. It is often a good way for the young doctor to gather some useful local intelligence. The first appraisal is often as useful for making a new local relationship as it is for any specific educational value. After your first one, however, you should be better clued up for the one the year after, at which stage the need for some evidence is much clearer.

RECORDING YOUR EVIDENCE FOR APPRAISAL

Unfortunately, the recording processes at present (April 2012) are far from fully clear. The ideal system would be an electronic toolkit that allowed you to record your information and your appraiser to see this information easily. Also, the local appraisal administrator would know the appraisal had happened (without seeing the full details of the appraisal content) and the responsible officer would be able to see the summaries of each appraisal. Obviously, such a system is not yet in place.

This ideal system would prompt the appraisee to record the basic facts about an event, and it would then give enough prompts to remind the appraisee to record their reflections and learning points from the event. Likewise, it would have similar prompts (nudges) for the other components: clinical audit, SEA, MSF, PF, complaint handling. The key is for the toolkit to record the learning event and then to help the appraisee show their reflection and thereby what they have learned from the event.

There are various toolkits available to record your appraisal (as listed earlier), so choose whichever one suits your style.

SCHEDULING APPRAISALS

Appraisal is an annual event, and you know it is coming up. You should know that having an annual appraisal is part of your obligations if you are to stay on the performers list. Despite this, many GPs are still surprised when their appraiser contacts them to set a date for the appraisal. This has led to a phenomenon in which although the appraisal year ran from April to March, over half of the appraisals were squeezed into the busiest time of the year between January and March. In the Calderdale area we have moved to scheduling appraisals by month of birth. This means that those who have an April birthday know their appraisal will be in April and so forth. It makes our appraisal year run much more smoothly, and it spreads the work over the year. Many other areas are adopting similar strategies; these strategies are better for both appraisers and appraisees.

CHOOSING YOUR APPRAISER

Most primary care trusts have a list of several appraisers. Sometimes you may be allocated to an appraiser whom you do not like for some reason. If this happens then you can ask for another appraiser (via the local appraisal administrator).

Now, if you have one person you do not like and you request a change, fair enough. However, if you pick problems with all the appraisers on the primary care trust's list, then it is more likely that it is you who have the problem.

Should you choose a hawk or a dove appraiser? Like examiners, some appraisers are thought softer and some harder. In practice it probably does not matter much; what matters is the work you put into preparing for the appraisal – it *is* *your* appraisal, isn't it? The appraisal is all about *you*, not the appraiser. The key thing is that you can have a useful formative and developmental conversation with your appraiser. Beware some doves seem gentle but they may actually be scathingly insightful; conversely, many hawks are not as threatening as they seem.

As a general rule, accept whomever you get allocated to do your appraisal unless there is some specific interpersonal problem.

WEAKNESSES OF THE APPRAISAL SYSTEM

There are some significant weaknesses to the appraisal system. The first of these is a cognitive flaw we all have: we tend to gild the lily in areas we already know well and miss the gaps in our knowledge of other areas. In appraisal, the appraisee presents positive evidence of what they have done and why, and the appraiser properly pays attention to this. What goes unsaid by the appraisee, and most times unnoticed by the appraiser, is where the areas of weakness and ignorance lie.

Very few of us are aware of our areas of ignorance. If we were, we would have done something about them! Appraisal does not have a system within it to pick up on these.[10-12] The RCGP toolkit has its inbuilt 'curriculum coverage' feature. This allows doctors to categorise their learning in terms of the RCGP curriculum for GP registrars. As the curriculum does not alter in medicine – the patients and their diseases are the same, whatever stage of medical practice you are at – then this feature allows you to see which areas have lots of CPD entries and which have none. If used conscientiously and consistently, this system could provide a way of spotting what we have not already considered in our CPD.

Second, appraisal can become a cosy chat, lacking challenge or focus. There can be collusion between the appraiser and the appraisee. Many appraisal systems change the appraiser every 2–3 years to prevent this from happening. The evidence requirements are not all that specific, and it is possible to get away with presenting some fairly poor-quality or minimal evidence to the appraiser. When area-wide statistical evidence such as commissioning data is presented, it is doubtful that most doctors are good enough at understanding statistics to fully grasp its meaning, or their personal contribution to the whole.

Third, appraisal is very poor at detecting poor performance. In other industries[12] appraisal is very much a performance review, but in medicine appraisal is at best partially effective at this. Appraisal is good at providing positive evidence that some sort of CPD process is being followed, and the assumption is that if a doctor is pursuing CPD then they are showing conscientious concern about their performance. The inference is that a doctor who neglects his or her CPD is a poor one. However, most medical directors say that they become aware of poorly performing doctors through routes other than appraisal.[13] To a large extent, appraisal is the nice bit of the local clinical governance processes – the bit that confirms to the medical director that people are doing the right things.

Despite its limitations, appraisal is the best process we have developed so far for ensuring ongoing CPD and support for doctors by doctors. It is an opportunity, and it is worth making as much of this opportunity as you can.

HOW TO FAIL YOUR APPRAISAL

You cannot fail your appraisal, but you can create trouble for yourself by failing to engage with the process (e.g. by not speaking to your appraiser, or by providing no evidence for the appraisal).

Remember that appraisal is a contractual obligation, and that refusing to take part in it allows the medical director to justify opening performers list proceedings against you very easily. If you lose your performers list status you will have a struggle to get it back again, in either your current or another primary care trust area.

As a doctor you would be silly not to engage with the appraisal process – it is mostly harmless, it can even be enjoyable, and you might learn something from it. Catching the medical director's attention for the wrong reasons is not sensible.

REFERENCES

1 General Medical Council. *GMP Framework for Appraisal and Revalidation*. GMC; 2011. Available at: www.gmc-uk.org/doctors/revalidation/revalidation_gmp_framework.asp (accessed 17 December 2011).

2 Royal College of General Practitioners. *Revalidation*. Available at: www.rcgp.org.uk/revalidation.aspx (accessed 17 December 2011).

3 Vincent C. *Patient Safety*. 2nd ed. West Sussex: Wiley-Blackwell; 2010.

4 Haynes K, Thomas M. *Clinical Risk Management in Primary Care*. Oxford: Radcliffe Publishing; 2005.

5 National Patient Safety Agency. *Significant Event Audit*. London: NPSA; 2008. Available at: www.nrls.npsa.nhs.uk/resources/?entryid45=61500 (accessed 17 December 2011).

6 Senge P. *The Fifth Discipline: the art and practice of the learning organisation*. London: Century Business; 1990.

7 Goldsmith M. *What Got You Here Won't Get You There: how successful people become even more successful*. London: Profile Books; 2008.

8 Eve R. *PUNs and DENs: discovering learning needs in general practice.* Oxford: Radcliffe Publishing; 2003.

9 Schon D. *The Reflective Practitioner: how professionals think in action.* Aldershot: Ashgate Publishing; 1991.

10 Schulz K. *Being Wrong: adventures in the margin of error.* London: Portobello Books; 2010.

11 Kruger J, Dunning D. Unskilled and unaware of it: how difficulties in recognizing one's own incompetence lead to inflated self-assessments. *J Pers Soc Psychol.* 1999; 77(6): 1121–34.

12 Coens T, Jenkins M. *Abolishing Performance Appraisals: why they backfire and what to do instead.* San Francisco: Berrett-Koehler Publishers; 2002.

13 Cox SJ, Holden JD. Presentation and outcome of clinical poor performance in one health district over a 5-year period: 2002–2007. *Br J Gen Pract.* 2009; **59**(562): 344–8.

D Personal development plans

Peter Davies

Your decisions about your CPD activity are usually crystallised by creating and maintaining a personal development plan (PDP). The appraiser will review progress under the revalidation headings and against the previous year's PDP goals. This progress is documented as part of the appraisal summary document (Form 4).

There is an art to setting PDP goals. They need to be interesting enough to be worth doing, but not so large that they are unattainable. Some GPs need tiny, baby-step goals, and some are only interested when the goals are large enough to be interesting. For example, if I had told my appraiser last year that I was going to write this book he would have said, 'That's a huge goal, Peter. Shouldn't you break it up into smaller steps?' Actually, my co-authors and I have just got on and written it, and it's nowhere on our PDPs at all! At some stage I will have to drag myself back to my PDP.

PDP goals are supposed to be SMART – that is, specific, measurable, achievable, realistic and time-bound. Sometimes the goals are set as small, miserable, average, all too realistic and timid; sometimes they are stupendous, magnificent, awesome, revelatory and tremendous. For most doctors, keeping them somewhere between the extremes is sensible. There is a lot to be said for making them achievable, even though I suspect this makes them lack much stretch or stimulus for many appraisees. Jennings[1] reviews this area thoroughly, and questions how well PDP goals match how we work out what we actually need to learn.

Ideally, PDP goals are suggested by the appraisee and confirmed and refined with the appraiser. As an appraiser there is nothing worse than encountering an appraisee who makes no positive suggestions and expects you to come up with a ready-made plan for them. It results in irrelevant, boring PDP goals that are often ignored.

The number of PDP goals you need is variable, depending on the doctor and their identified educational needs. The usual recommendation is between three and six goals. Ideally the goals should be personal. Sometimes a doctor has a goal that is actually a project they can only complete by involving the whole practice – for example, to construct a practice business plan. It is not clear whether this should count as a personal or a practice development goal.

Goals that involve many people, conversations and meetings are intrinsically harder to achieve, but they may actually be what is needed at practice level. As yet there is no system of practice development and practice appraisal. However, as an appraiser I often feel that what I am seeing in one appraisee's folder is an issue that needs to go to the whole practice team, but as an appraiser I can only deal with the individual doctor . . . and there is a tension here.

For appraisal personal development plan goals, keeping them within your own sphere of action and influence is more sensible, on the whole. Also, remember that, in terms of Stephen Covey's model of spheres of action,[2] the more effective you are within your sphere of action the greater becomes your sphere of influence, and so the greater your eventual impact on your sphere of concern.

REFERENCES

1 Jennings SF. Personal development plans and self-directed learning for healthcare professionals: are they evidence based? *Postgrad Med J.* 2007; **83**(982): 518–24.
2 Covey S. *The 7 Habits of Highly Effective People.* Reprint. New York: Simon & Schuster; 2004.

E Revalidation

Peter Davies

Revalidation is basically a mechanism for making sure that your professional life is keeping on track, with you maintaining your sanity and the patients benefiting from rather than harmed by your interventions. This is officially phrased as showing that you are 'fit for purpose and up to date'. It has specific requirements and mechanisms that are still being finalised. The details are found in the *RCGP Guide to Revalidation* on the RCGP website[1] and in the responsible officer regulations.[2] The RCGP document is a work in progress and it is updated regularly so you are best to consult it at the time you want to see what exactly you need to do.

When it was first mooted, revalidation seemed like a major threat and challenge to many doctors. It appeared that it was going to be a complex, high-stakes examination that could end up with many doctors failing it and being referred to fitness to practise panels at the General Medical Council (GMC). Estimates of between 5% and 15% of doctors having to go through this ordeal were mentioned. As there are about 240 000 GMC-registered doctors, that could have meant 2500–5000 GMC referrals per year just from revalidation. Apart from anything else, the GMC just does not have enough capacity for so much extra activity. As a senior colleague of mine commented, 'It's like medical finals – they cannot fail us all at once – they wouldn't have anyone left to do the work next year.'

Revalidation is now becoming a more minor presence. Our licences to practise now have a time limit on them of 5 years, after which they need to be revalidated. For most of us this will be about as interesting a process as renewing a library book. However, it is important as it allows you to maintain your licence to practise intact, which is a precious asset.

If you are part of a well-functioning clinical governance system that has no current concerns about you and you have completed all your appraisals at least to a reasonable standard, then the responsible officer (RO) (who may well be the local medical director) has no option but to recommend you for revalidation. If you have a special circumstance such as an unresolved complaint or you have been on prolonged ill-health leave, then the decision will be to defer revalidation until a specified date in the future. This postpones the decision, and leaves intact your licence to practise.

If you fail totally to engage with continuing professional development, appraisal and revalidation processes then you are likely to be perpetrating serious professional misconduct and therefore risk a referral through to the GMC.

If you have given the medical director cause for concern about your fitness to practise sufficient to make him or her reach the threshold for referral to the GMC, then they will already have made that referral on the evidence available at the time. That decision will have been made a long time prior to the revalidation decision. You will already know about it. There will be no 'sudden unexpected failures' at revalidation. Such an event would be seen as a major failure of the local clinical governance processes.

You will not be able to fail revalidation, and it is not a process designed to get more doctors into the GMC fitness to practise procedures.

Revalidation cannot take your licence to practise away from you – only a GMC fitness to practise panel can do that. For most doctors it will be a minor event, emerging from local clinical governance processes working well.

Although the formal decision to revalidate lies with the GMC, in practice they are not looking to overturn the recommendations they will receive from the local ROs, so effectively the process is mostly locally based. Currently it looks as if there will be one RO for each primary care trust cluster area.

Whether this process has much merit to it is debated and the review by Greenhalgh and Wong[3] is worth reading. A more positive spin is presented in a later paper.[4]

THE RESPONSIBLE OFFICER

It is not worth a GP, young or old, worrying much about who their RO is. The connections from individual doctors to their responsible officers are defined by the GMC and described on their website. The work of the RO is very procedurally bound.[2] That is, the RO has little discretion about the revalidation decisions he or she can make; therefore, it does not much matter for you as individual GP who the RO is.

Where there is a potential or actual conflict of interest between the RO and the doctor whose performance he or she is reviewing, then another RO (probably from a neighbouring area or a deputy RO) will act in his or her place.

I HAVE MY REVALIDATION COMING UP: WHAT DO I NEED TO DO?

Relax, send the required information in, and wait for the RO to confirm that you should be revalidated. Seriously, you should know the outcome of the revalidation decision before it is made. There should be no surprises about it. It is entirely a process- and rule-based decision. There is no room for personal opinion, and the RO is simply applying the rules, which are well published and publicised.

If you heading towards failing revalidation you should know about this long before it gets to revalidation day. Although revalidation is an event that occurs once every 5 years, it reflects processes running throughout the 5 years, and unlike medical finals you cannot cram it all in the last month. As long as you have participated in the appraisal process, produced the evidence needed and answered any complaints sensibly, then the RO has to revalidate you.

However, if you have avoided appraisal, done little learning, and not paid attention to your appraiser's hints, then you may encounter trouble at revalidation time. This would not be the fault of the process: it would be your failure to engage with it intelligently. It is likely the RO would have had concerns about you a long while prior to the revalidation decision and already acted on them.

REFERENCES

1 Royal College of General Practitioners. *Guide to Revalidation*. Available at: www. rcgp.org.uk/pdf/Guide%20to%20Revalidation%20for%20GPs_sixth_edn_210911. pdf (accessed 12 March 2012).

2 National Archives. *The Medical Profession (Responsible Officers) Regulations 2010*. Available at: www.legislation.gov.uk/uksi/2010/2841/made (accessed 17 December 2011).

3 Greenhalgh T, Wong G. Revalidation: a critical perspective. *Br J Gen Pract*. 2011; **61**(584): 166–8.

4 Davies P, Walsh M, Pollock C. Performance management, appraisals, and revalidation: quantity analysis and quality control for UK GPs. *Br J Gen Pract*. 2011; **61**(589): 526–7.

F Clinical governance

Peter Davies

In each area there are now increasingly well-described clinical governance processes that describe what will be done if a doctor's performance gives cause for concern.

Basically there are two channels in operation:
1. the one that you want (**the learning channel** – continuing professional development (CPD), appraisal, demonstrating your pride and commitment to lifelong learning and development)
2. the one that you want to avoid as far as possible (**the clinical governance** system – complaints, serious incidents, outlying performance, other causes for concern).

None of us will totally avoid complaints and it is worth being polite and respectful to the local complaints officer. He or she has a difficult job and is often getting it in the neck from patients. If you convince him or her that you are just as bad as the patient has said you are, then you may be making your troubles worse than they need to be!

The General Medical Council (GMC) describes a four-layer model of professional regulation:
1. the doctor's professional conscience
2. the doctor's immediate colleagues
3. the local regulatory processes (primary care trust, and likely the NHS Commissioning Board in future)
4. the national regulatory processes (i.e. the GMC).

The GMC has often lamented that local clinical governance processes were scanty and underdeveloped and that it was involved in cases that should have been sorted out locally. The GMC is interested in cases of 'serious professional misconduct' and the word serious here implies either sustained poor performance or a particularly bad example of poor performance. In this context the thresholds are high, and ordinary mistakes, minor complaints and even most negligence actions fall below it. A new development is the network of employment liaison advisors being set up by the GMC to liaise with medical directors about doctors giving cause for concern.

There is now a developing network of primary care medical directors who have a specific interest in management of performance issues. In each area there are now well-described routes of investigation and judgement of doctors who give cause for concern. The separation of investigation from decision-making is very important.

How do medical directors come to know about a doctor whose conduct is a cause for concern? The main routes for medical directors coming to know about a doctor whose conduct is a cause for concern are:

- complaints
- serious untoward incidents
- criminal convictions
- outlying clinical behaviours (e.g. high prescribing, excessive referrals).[1]

Medical directors are not looking for trouble, but they will tackle it when they find it. It is to be hoped that clinical governance will not be something that many have to encounter and there are ways to avoid this potentially unpleasant route.

If you do come under a 'cause for concern' investigation then the following advice may help reduce the damage. You do not want additional casualties, or more broken relationships than necessary. Cooperate with the investigation, accept an occupational health assessment, show that you are learning something from the experience. Follow your medical director's and medical defence organisation's advice to the letter. If you want to swear, do it privately; in public be politeness personified.

Get whatever support you need from colleagues, occupational health and the medical defence teams.

SUMMARY

When you leave your vocational training scheme and move onto a performers list you come under the umbrella of the local clinical governance processes. These basically have two sides to them.

1. There's a 'good cop': your conscience, your licence to practise, your CPD, your appraisal and appraisers, the educational system. This recognises, records, supports and encourages your positive contributions.
2. There's a 'bad cop': complaints, outlying performance, criminal convictions, clinical governance concerns, the medical director in his or her investigatory role. This shows when your actions have become a negative contribution.

Provided you talk to the good cop and you don't trigger the bad cop's concerns, you get revalidated. Revalidation is basically a routine output from your local clinical governance and educational/appraisal processes.

Your licence to practise medicine is vital to you. It needs to be maintained, and the maintenance is done by means of CPD confirmed at appraisal. Try to stay clear of the clinical governance and performance processes. If you can achieve these two things then your revalidation is sorted.

Medical directors are best known as intelligent and respected senior colleagues, rather than encountered in an investigation.

REFERENCE

1 Cox SJ, Holden JD. Presentation and outcome of clinical poor performance in one health district over a 5-year period: 2002–2007. *Br J Gen Pract*. 2009; **59**(562): 344–8.

Chapter **8**

Leadership

Peter Davies, with input from Lindsay Moran

If your actions inspire others to dream more, learn more, do more and become more, you are a leader.

—John Quincy Adams

Readers are leaders.

—John Maxwell

Everyone who's ever taken a shower has an idea. It's the person who gets out of the shower, dries off and does something about it who makes a difference.

—Nolan Bushnell

No institution can possibly survive if it needs geniuses or supermen to manage it. It must be organized in such a way as to be able to get along under a leadership composed of average human beings.

—Peter Drucker

Leadership must be based on goodwill. Goodwill does not mean posturing and, least of all, pandering to the mob. It means obvious and wholehearted commitment to helping followers. We are tired of leaders we fear, tired of leaders we love, and of tired of leaders who let us take liberties with them. What we need for leaders are men of the heart who are so helpful that they, in effect, do away with the need of their jobs. But leaders like that are never out of a job, never out of followers. Strange as it sounds, great leaders gain authority by giving it away.

—Admiral James B Stockdale

Great leaders are almost always great simplifiers, who can cut through argument, debate, and doubt to offer a solution everybody can understand.

—General Colin Powell

Keep away from people who belittle your ambitions. Small people always do that, but the really great make you feel that you, too, can become great.

—Mark Twain

Success consists of getting up just one more time than you fall.

—Oliver Goldsmith

INTRODUCTION

In this chapter, and Chapter 9 on commissioning, we move into some fascinating, contentious and contested territory.

At present in the NHS there is a crying need for leadership. Commissioning is the newest leadership task coming to GPs and as it is such a large topic and so topical it takes up a chapter of its own. However, remember that the profession needs leadership in many other areas and tasks and at many levels. For example, your training programme directors have been leading your education on your vocational training scheme. Many roles in medicine involve taking a lead; that lead starts from the leads you give to your patients, and it moves up through all the levels of medical effectiveness to the lead someone like Clare Gerada gives to our specialty in her role as RCGP chair of council. In short, leadership is intrinsic to our work as doctors.

Followership is also intrinsic to our work. We (GPs) cannot all lead everything, and all of us have to accept at least some leadership from others at various times. We are none of us complete as individuals, and we need to know who to follow and why we choose to follow them and not someone else. At any time we are all leading and we are all following. Whether we are leading our partner gracefully on the dance floor or leading our partners a merry dance in the surgery, someone is leading and someone is following. We are all taking and giving cues, to ourselves and to others, all the time. We are all seeking to influence and persuade other people to do something else. As Aristotle rightly said, 'man is by nature a political animal'. We are all trying to influence those we meet, moving them towards something and away from other things.

So the questions then become, 'How do we lead well?' and 'How do we follow well?' How should we join in the processes of leading and following well and to our own and other people's benefit?

WHAT MAKES A GOOD LEADER?

When you consider the various qualities of leaders from both the present and the past, you can pick out a number of attributes that set them aside from the followers – these are often more obvious in retrospect. Think how many MPs get cursed with being labelled as 'the next prime minister but three' and then get sent out to govern New South Wales.[1]

Leaders vary in their styles and personalities: some are extrovert, others introvert; some like to rule with dominance and are dictatorial; others rule with democracy and are decision enablers rather than decision enforcers.

Some qualities attributable to leaders can include:
- good team-working skills
- confidence
- passion for their role
- good communicators
- good orators
- analysis and problem-solving skills
- persuasive and influencing
- people and task management skills
- vision
- resilience
- flexibility
- good motivators.

When we think of leaders though, there are some names that commonly jump out at us: Barack Obama, Nelson Mandela, Sir Winston Churchill, Mohandas Gandhi, the Queen, Angela Merkel, Steve Jobs, Princess Diana, Pope John Paul II, Margaret Thatcher and the list goes on. The list of most mentioned leaders alters over time and shows a 'currency' effect – we remember those who are currently in the news rather than the full cast of history. Where is Vice-Admiral Nelson on that list? Or Edward the First?

There are other leaders who, despite in their prime having commanded an enormous following and having been hugely influential and powerful, history has taken a negative view of because of their excessive wielding of power, their eccentricities and their killing of thousands to millions of their opposition. These leaders include the likes of Hitler, Stalin, Mugabe, Gaddafi and Saddam Hussein. Even though these leaders abused their power, the fact remains that they were able to influence and lead millions of people.

In other words, leadership skills are useful, but it is even more important that we remember the end they are directed towards, and that leadership skills are only a means towards this.

When we consider any leader we tend to find that they had great success, often built on many failures, and no apparent direction when younger. Think of Churchill's early career and its many disasters. Yet he was right about one big thing, and so became our great wartime prime minister.[2] Equally, he was a leader for that season of our national life but was dumped unceremoniously at the end of the Second World War when his task was complete.

Sometimes the supreme act of leadership is to recognise when your time has passed, and not to go on and on. Fixed-term appointments, such as 3 years as chair of council or a maximum 8 years (two terms) as president of the United States, help with this.

There is a huge literature about leadership and strategies and we recommend the books listed at the end of this chapter as a route into this field. Strangely, there is a dearth of information about followership, yet for most people knowing who and what to follow is more important than leading.

GOOD EXAMPLES AND DIRE WARNINGS

The key when considering leaders is to realise that they all have both good points and flaws. Try to learn from the good points and reduce the flaws. Unfortunately, this balance of good points and flaws applies to all of us, and sometimes it is our flaws that propel us into leadership roles. Equally commonly, our fears and false modesties often keep us away from leadership roles that we could in fact do very well. Remember that here fear is an acronym for 'false evidence appearing real'. Don't live down to your own misunderestimation of yourself.

SOME GENERAL FRAMES OF REFERENCE AROUND LEADERSHIP

> *Who sets the frame sets the game.*
>
> —Richard Bandler

I need now to describe some general frames around leadership and show you how much your own life has been and still is being led by others. As you grow in the profession and in life generally I hope you will become more conscious of the lead you are giving or not giving and of the people and things you agree to follow or are forced to follow by system default.

As a medical student and then as a young doctor you have been educated within a curriculum that is a frame of reference that defines what you need to know to get through your course. You have accepted this frame of reference, partially because you had to and partially because when you filled in your Universities and Colleges Admissions Service form and medical training applications you chose to accept a certain path in life and to thereby exclude certain other courses of action. You have trusted your educators and examiners to know what you need to know and have accepted the frames of reference they have laid down around your learning and thinking for many years. Before medical school you had mostly accepted the frames of reference laid down by parents and teachers, mainly because you had to – you would not have known enough to completely set your own course in life. You may have rebelled as a teenager but if you did so it was probably with no clear idea of what you were against or what you were for.

So, you have largely accepted a follower role in the early part of your life.

You will still be a follower for much of your professional life. For example, as a GP, I now do PHQ9 (Patient Health Questionnaire) scores to attempt to quantify the severity of the depression my patient is suffering from.[3] This is an external imposition onto my style of medicine having everything to do with how I am paid (via the quality and outcomes framework (QOF)) and little to do with any medicine I know or personal wish for improvement. There is a more general argument as to whether or not condition-specific questionnaires improve the accuracy of clinical assessment or not, but I, like most GPs, have not used them very much in practice.[4] So, in my use of the PHQ9 scores I am following the external and imposed leadership of the QOF, which believes that GPs will assess depression better if they use a scoring system rather than just their clinical nous. My motives for accepting the imposition are largely venial (to get paid) rather than clinical.

There is an element of me thinking, 'well, if that is what they will pay me for then that is what I will do.' Also, there is pressure from my partners to make sure we all meet QOF targets so that we all get paid. Margaret Thatcher once commented that 'you can't buck the market'. In the consulting room maybe we can't buck our incentives. It does not feel like great medicine, but it is how the system makes it.

COGNITIVE DISSONANCE: THE DRIVER FOR LEADERSHIP?

Some doctors just accept this kind of thing and keep their head down, working away quietly within a system that gets progressively madder the more clearly you come to see it. Others experience cognitive dissonance, a sense that 'this isn't right', and they get annoyed enough to wish to do something about it. I do not believe that anything alters until someone (a person – I hope it is you, not a committee, not a college, not any of the great collective 'they') gets annoyed enough to act. Somewhere inside each of us there is an issue that will propel us past our tipping point[5] and into action. The issue in fact creates your opportunity.

Once you have reached this point then you are moving into becoming a clinical leader – someone who does something about things that are wrong, as opposed to someone who merely whinges. Remember that whinges are very common but people willing to do anything about these whinges are far fewer.

Maybe clinical leadership should be seen as the creative transformation of whinges and glitches into free-flowing systems of care.

At this stage you may not be very experienced or strategic about how to instigate change. Your contribution at this stage may be more enthusiastic than skilful. Don't worry about this; rather, show willingness, talk to colleagues, gather allies and see what emerges.

WHERE IS CLINICAL LEADERSHIP NEEDED?

Clinical leadership is needed throughout the NHS. There is only one thing worse than participating in the processes of clinical leadership and that is to stay on the sideline and see someone less intelligent and less experienced than yourself making a hash of things.

The main venues for clinical leadership are as follows:
- of patients in the consulting room
- of colleagues in the practice
- in education and training
- in the appraisal systems
- in clinical commissioning groups
- in guideline development
- in specialised bodies (e.g. primary care societies)
- in British Medical Association, local medical committee and RCGP faculties
- in local system service improvements.

You can make a choice to not be involved in leadership, but your personal and professional life will be poorer for such a choice. It will be poorer in terms of knowledge, relationship building, effectiveness, understanding and appreciation of others and why they act as they do. Your personal power will reduce as you try to retreat within yourself and 'just keep on doing the work'.

At some stage of your career you have to start to lead or others will lead you. If you decline the challenge then you will be taken by others in directions you may not want to go, with no say about where you are going and why. At some point later in your career you will start to bleat about 'lots of stress' and 'burnout' and 'disempowerment' and 'this isn't what I trained for' and 'those idiots in their ivory towers who just don't know how hard it is being a GP in the poorer end of Greater Cleckhuddersfax'. Meanwhile, you the doctor who actually knows what needs to be done will become increasingly frustrated that no one is doing it. This is because YOU SHOULD BE DOING IT!

For example, in my own experience in Calderdale we had a problem with X-rays and the time it took for results to come back to GPs.[6] I would send a patient with an X-ray card to the local hospital and the pictures would be taken quickly, and the radiologists were doing their job well and reporting all films within 24 hours. Yet, despite this, the radiographers would tell the patients that 'the results will be with your GP in 2 weeks'. I would regularly have consultations that went along the lines of the patients asking, 'Has the X-ray result come back yet? They said it would be here by now', and I would despair and say, 'They may have said that, but they never get here that quickly'. The patient had wasted his or her time and energy and I had had a largely wasted consultation; the result would finally limp into the surgery 3 or 4 weeks, and one or two wasted appointments, later. A piece of paper had taken several weeks to travel the 4 miles between my surgery and the hospital. In the same time I had sent a paper to a journal in the United States and it had been reviewed and accepted. Everything inside me said that this was wrong, so I nagged away at the primary care trust and hospital chief executives. I pointed out that the problem I saw was:

- common
- wasting patient time
- adding needlessly to patient worry
- potentially risky to patient safety and service reputation
- wasting doctor time, and reducing our accessibility by wasting appointments
- squandering money.

The local medical committee gave me support in this campaign. What was remarkable about this process was that there are 130 GPs on the performers list in Calderdale and only two or three of us raised any noise about the issue. Most of my colleagues (who were just as aware of this problem as I was) said nothing about it.

Eventually, meetings were convened to look at the problem I had identified, and from solutions emerged from this process. Having nagged so much, I was in honour bound to work with this process. We now have electronic requesting and reporting of X-rays and scans. Now I am disappointed and surprised if the result is not available within a few days, and when I see patients for results the results are available and I can explain their meaning to the patient, rather than moaning about delays in the system. In other words, the system now lets me do the useful medicine well to help patients, rather than all of us simply getting frustrated.

In your own area and practice you may well have a similar problem that needs sorting. Please do something about it. The patients deserve the decent service, not a succession of glitches, and you are probably good at medicine and bad at glitches.

HOW DO I GET INVOLVED IN CLINICAL LEADERSHIP?

You will not be able to avoid all leadership in your career, even if you just keep it within your own surgery, and some of you reading this will eventually move up through the ranks and move to local, regional and national leadership positions. There is a process to go through to get ready for such development.

There are many ways to get into leadership in our profession. The first way is to **show willingness and turn up**. This is an apprenticeship-type model, but if you attend voluntarily, and then get elected onto (and paid to be on) your local medical committee it is a good start. Alternatively, many RCGP faculty boards need young volunteers. Could you lead some educational events for them? Maybe aimed at students or your fellow new GPs? In this sort of forum you meet existing leaders, you can see their good and bad points, and you can develop your own style over time. You can see how arguments get framed and presented, and which arguments prove persuasive and which fall by the wayside. You can hide in the body, and learn a lot by watching, and then gradually move to start contributing yourself. You probably won't get the big papers and topics to lead on at first. However, all papers need checking and proofreading – could you help the more senior leader with that process?

Sometimes there are vacancies going begging at the primary care trust – for example, in Halifax we had not had a protected learning time tutor for some time and our monthly educational meeting called 'PENPALs' had been struggling. What vacancy is going begging in your local organisations? Could you help your local colleagues by taking it? I have seen bright young doctors grab such an opportunity and make a lot of it and therefore come to be seen as senior colleagues before they reach the age of 40.

The clinical commissioning groups are going to need clinical help and engagement on specific topics. Clinical commissioning group board members are working at a strategic level, and to do this they are going to need well worked up information about current provision, relevant evidence and national standards and guidelines, and recommendations for action. There is going to be a need for other doctors to help their board members by getting this information together for them. Could you help them by gathering this information? And maybe learn a fair bit yourself in the process? This could well be paid project-type work. It may be a good place for you to start.

Perhaps you want to teach undergraduate students. It can be a great starting point for a teaching portfolio.

Perhaps you want to know more about what the lead or senior partner does – if so, show interest and ask questions. Perhaps there is a project at the surgery that needs doing? Could you do it? Or perhaps you and one of the other partners? I bet the other partners would be very grateful if you did it. All the while you complete this work your reputation and credibility is building.

Perhaps you pioneer a new project – I think of the bravery of my friend Dr Nat Wright as he led the development of a new service to the homeless in Leeds.

I can think of some younger GPs who have taken over a single-handed practice that looks a bit run down and through hard work and intelligence got it up to a high clinical and training standard. Such characters get a lot of respect.

As you can see, there are many places from which you can start, and to be honest the great point here is simply to start. As Goethe stated, 'Whatever you can do or dream you can, begin it. Boldness has genius, power and magic in it.'

The second way is through **taught courses** – there are many available. They can help your development, but you are often better to be learning by experience first, so that the theory and the practice begin to join together. One way of getting a good overview of the opportunities for leadership is to take a taught masters degree in primary care. These courses are often excellent and are a good way to meet many people and learn a lot from the work, the academic faculty and your colleagues on the course. These courses introduce you to the great conversations going on within and around primary care and show you how they are structured and how they work.

The third way is through **personal reading**. There is extensive literature available about leadership and it has much of value within it. I have suggested a starting list at the end of the chapter. As a general rule, and as John Maxwell describes, 'readers become leaders'. If personal reading is combined with reflection on the good examples and dire warnings you have seen in your medical and personal life, you can come to see how some leaders do it well and how some do it badly. Personal reading combined with reflection on experience has much to recommend it, and it adds to the other strategies you are using.

Research can be a way into leadership positions, either as an academic or in service development settings. If your research is genuinely taking us to see new or different horizons then you are inevitably leading away from the status quo and into a new and hopefully better possibility.

There are many ways into medical leadership, but availability, intelligence, knowledge and reflection are usually key components, whichever part of the game you end up playing. Also, some degree of patience, keeping an eye on the medium to long term, some resilience, some humour, and an ability to understand how the world looks to somebody else are all useful points. You learned most of these things as consultation skills – they work pretty well in leadership contexts too.

In essence, doctors all have the opportunity to be leaders for their patients, communities and peers. How far each person takes that role is an individual matter, but with adherence to good leadership qualities and vision there is always scope for positive change.

FOLLOWERSHIP

There is much talk about leadership in the NHS, but there is also a need for some people to be followers. We cannot all lead everything. So most of us will be sometimes leading and sometimes following. You may not want to be a leader, but it is well worth deciding who and what you want to follow. If you know this, you will be able to justify your thoughts and actions well. If you do not, the many passing fancies and guidelines that come and go will blow you about. You will end up serving the transient and you will lose your focus on what actually matters; by mid-career you will be bewildered.

If you are going to follow people and ideas, please do this wholeheartedly and without too much whinging – it is to be hoped that your leaders will justify your trust and respect.

There is a balance between leading and following that alters throughout our careers and it is worthwhile knowing where you are on this balance. I hope that in this chapter I have given some useful pointers about leadership in general, and in our NHS context. In the next chapter I will describe commissioning, which is the biggest current leadership challenge facing our specialty.

REFERENCES

1 Belloc H. Lord Lundy. In: *Cautionary Tales for Children*. 1907. Available at: http://theotherpages.org/poems/belloc02.html (accessed 17 December 2011).
2 Gilbert M. *Churchill: a life*. London: Pimlico; 2000.
3 Leydon GM, Dowrick CF, McBride AS, *et al*. Questionnaire severity measures for depression: a threat to the doctor-patient relationship? *Br J Gen Pract*. 2011; **61**(583): 117–23.
4 Jenkinson C. *Health Status Measurement*. Oxford: Radcliffe Medical Press; 1998.
5 Gladwell M. *The Tipping Point: how little things can make a big difference*. London: Abacus; 2002.
6 Davies P. The great NHS communication breakdown. *BMJ*. 2008; **337**(7662): 176.

FURTHER READING

There is a huge literature around leadership and organisational development. The books here are favourites of mine, and I think they provide a good introduction to the leadership literature. Once you become interested in this area the field opens up significantly.

- Carnegie D. *How to Win Friends and Influence People*. Kingswood, Tadworth, Surrey: World's Work (1913) Ltd; 1953. Remember everyone's name and so on.
- Cialdini R. *Influence: science and practice*. Boston, MA: Allyn & Bacon; 2001. A great book showing how we give and receive influence. Worth reading both to use yourself and to enjoy spotting the methods that other people use on you.
- Colvin G. *Talent is Overrated: what* really *separates world-class performers from everybody else*. London: Nicholas Brealey Publishing; 2008. A book about how to get really good at any activity – 10,000 hours of focused practice seems to be the answer.
- Katzenbach JR, Garvin DA, Etienne C. *Harvard Business Review on Teams that Succeed*. Boston, MA: Harvard Business Publishing; 2004. The story about the Nut Island disaster is a superb account of technical versus managerial ways of knowing, and of where the sewage ends up when they talk past each other.
- Kay J. *Obliquity: why our goals are best achieved indirectly*. New York: Penguin; 2010. Points out the perils of a too direct approach to life – we don't always really know our starting point or where we want to get to.
- Kouzes JM, Posner BZ. *Credibility: how leaders gain and lose it, why people demand it*. San Francisco: Jossey-Bass; 2011. A superb account of how credibility is gained and lost – simply described but rarely fully achieved by any of us, however much we would like to attain and retain it.
- Magee B. *The Story of Philosophy*. London: Dorling Kindersley; 1998. A superb summary of the great philosophers and their ideas.
- Owens DA. *Creative People Must Be Stopped! 6 Ways we kill innovation (without even trying)*. San Fransisco: Jossey-Bass; 2012. An excellent look at how innovation gets stopped – sometimes for good reason and sometimes not. If you want to be a leader or innovator this book will guide you around many pitfalls.
- Royal College of General Practitioners. *The Future General Practitioner: learning and teaching*. London: RCGP; 1972. Who sets the frame sets the game, and this particular framework has kept us guided for the last 40 years.
- Schulz K. *Being Wrong: adventures in the margins of error*. New York: Ecco; 2010. Cromwell once said, 'I pray you consider you may be mistaken'. This book invites us to consider how easily and how often we are mistaken.
- Seddon J. *Systems Thinking in the Public Sector: the failure of the reform regime . . . and a manifesto for a better way*. Axminster: Triarchy Press; 2008. Fixing the bits does not work – focusing on unit costs sends them up. A clear overview of the power of systems thinking.

- Senior B. *Organisational Change*. 2nd ed. London: Prentice Hall; 2002. A straight-forward management textbook.
- Tudor-Hart JT. *A New Kind of Doctor: the general practitioner's part in the health of the community*. London: Merlin Press; 1988. A superb vision of what general practice could be like.
- Whyte D. *The Heart Aroused*. New York: Bantam-Doubleday; 2002. A wonderful book about rediscovering your sense of wonder and belonging at work.
- Wilson K. *The Games Climbers Play*. London: Diadem Books; 1978. Climbing is all about whom you trust to lead and whom you trust to follow. In particular, try the pieces by Mike Thompson on being a high-altitude porter on an Everest expedition, and the excuses list by Dr Tom Patey in 'The art of climbing down gracefully'.

Chapter 9

Commissioning

Peter Davies, with input from Lindsay Moran

Whatever course you decide upon, there is always someone to tell you that you are wrong. There are always difficulties arising which tempt you to believe that your critics are right. To map out a course of action and follow it to an end requires courage.

—Ralph Waldo Emerson

Events, dear boy, events.

—Harold Macmillan, British prime minister, when asked what terrified him

[A]ll care necessary from the cradle to the grave.

—Aneurin Bevan

They need have no fear – no fear at all. I conceive it the function of the Ministry of Health to provide the medical profession with the best and most modern apparatus of medicine and to enable them freely to use it, in accordance with their training, for the benefit of the people of the country. Every doctor must be free to use that apparatus without interference from secular organizations. The individual citizen must be free to choose his doctor and the doctor must be able to treat his patient in conditions of inviolable privacy. I look upon the general practitioner as the most important man in the medical profession, but I hope – and I trust this will not be regarded as tendentious – that

we shall be able to organize a service which will take general prac-
titioners away from the isolation in which at present many of them
live and work, and that more group associations will be organized
amongst them.

—Aneurin Bevan, 1945

After all – I need not remind you of this – I am a Socialist, and, being
a Socialist, I believe in industrial democracy, and because I believe in
industrial democracy I believe that doctors as a profession must have
a greater and greater say in the management of their own services.

—Aneurin Bevan, 1945

Warning: the ideas in this chapter are controversial, and their final form is not worked out. In this chapter I try to present a reasonably balanced account of commissioning and how GPs relate to this. I am an elected member of the Calderdale Clinical Commissioning Group. What I say here I have written personally but informed by my experience of commissioning so far. I am more optimistic about the likely success of commissioning than many colleagues are.[1,2] As always, time will tell, but for now I think that what we are being asked to achieve for the NHS is worthwhile and achievable. If as GPs we succeed in this role then our value to the NHS is increased, and our status will rise as people acknowledge both our clinical and our economic acumen. There is a certain irony that Aneurin Bevan always wanted doctors to have a greater say in the management of their own services – and it may be a 'lower than vermin' Tory secretary of state for health who actually delivers this to us . . . and that we may not be entirely keen on taking the opportunity offered.

WHAT IS COMMISSIONING?

In the Department of Health (DH) guidance on commissioning,[3] commissioning in the NHS is the process by which a health service commissioner specifies what services it needs from its healthcare service providers. Specifically, the role of GP commissioners has been defined as follows:

- To be the advocate for patients and communities – securing a range of appropriate high-quality healthcare services for people in need.
- To be the custodian of taxpayers' money – this brings a requirement to secure best value in the use of resources.
- To be advocates for health and well-being, encouraging and enabling

individuals, families and communities to take responsibility for staying healthy and managing their health and conditions.

This is a good definition of commissioning, as it emphasises population need, quality and efficiency and focuses on prevention and patient responsibility. Whether all these worthy objectives can be obtained via a single policy or aligned with one another is debatable.

WHY DOES THE NEED FOR COMMISSIONING ARISE?

Some history

Commissioning is a function that has eluded the NHS ever since it was created in 1948. The nationalisation of the hospitals in 1948 also saw rather a fossilisation of the hospitals; the historic pattern and distribution of healthcare was not altered – it was just that new management came in.

The DH in relation to the NHS has always rather assumed that its job is to run the service rather than to determine what that service should be. So if you read the history of the NHS in the accounts of Charles Webster[4] or Rudolf Klein[5] you will find that most DH work has been about keeping existing services running and trying to reduce the unmet need, especially waiting lists, encountered by the service. Prof David Haslam,[6] a great GP writer, laments that 'schools and hospitals' is a shorthand that uses a venue as a shorthand for processes of healthcare and education, and ends up confusing a means of healthcare delivery, with healthcare delivery that could be achieved in many different ways.

Some economics

In a market system the signals of cost connect supply with demand and over time act so as to balance them. In a nationalised health service these cost signals are lost. The NHS has a single stream of revenue (taxation), a single channel of distribution (the DH to its regional and local representatives) and a single channel of delivery (NHS staff and services).

Despite this singularity the NHS is characterised by much variation within and among doctors, hospitals and outcomes.[7] Despite being a national system, the NHS encountered in practice is patchy, peculiar and parochial. 'You do know that they do things differently at St Elsewhere's, don't you?'

The NHS is unusual among healthcare systems in developed countries in many ways. Most systems in Europe have an element of funding from multiple sources: local tax, national tax, levy on employers and some user charges. Most systems in Europe are more regional or locally based, so that local politicians and local managers run local hospitals. In Europe the idea that a dropped bedpan would echo anywhere other than where it was dropped would be laughed at. In the UK's centralised service its echoes can be heard in the corridors of Whitehall. In the

UK the local health services have been removed totally from local government's jurisdiction, and placed under the control of centrally made local appointees.

In Europe there is decentralised delivery of healthcare with multiple different chains of providers, not a single monolithic monopoly. In the UK we have an extremely centralised NHS run from the centre, with a management that, as its chief executive Sir David Nicholson describes it, tends to look 'upwards and inwards' for its direction and inspiration, rather than 'sidewards and outwards to its local area'. The NHS has had a strong culture of 'central credit and local blame'. Its senior leaders (chief executives) have often had less job security and shorter average tenures than football managers. And they have nearly all been sacked by people higher up in the DH, not by their local patients or their local communities.

In short, the NHS has been an extremely centralised funder, distributor and purchaser of healthcare. Realising this, there has been an attempt since the early 1990s by successive secretaries of state for health to try to create an 'internal' or 'mimic' market within the NHS. This has been done to try to get some of the perceived efficiencies and clear incentives for the NHS that exist in a market. There has been a move to hospitals becoming semi-detached businesses called 'foundation trusts' that can raise revenue in ways other than through government grants. There has been a move away from block grants to 'payment by results' (which is actually payment by activity) paid for under a tariff system that pays a sum of money for each item of work completed (e.g. a hip replacement).

There is an incentive under payment-by-results rules for a hospital to maximise its activity and do as much chargeable work as possible. The counterbalance to this was supposed to be the commissioning process vaingloriously described as 'world class commissioning',[8] which was to be led by primary care trusts with GPs involved via a process called 'practice-based commissioning'. Needless to say, these processes were failures[9] and have now been reworked and renamed. (It's a good rule in British public life that if you need to rename something it is not working, and it is unlikely to work any better under its new name.)

THE ECONOMICS IN THE GP'S SURGERY

For many of us seeing patients in our consultations is our primary concern. We prescribe and we refer in our patient's best interests. However, there is a need for us as doctors to own the economic impact as well as the clinical outcomes of their work.[10] There is a need for us to move on from just spending the system's resources and then shroud waving (the gaining of publicity by casting a blame over tragedy) when they run out. There is a need for us to acknowledge that our daily medical activity in our consulting rooms is both economic and clinical – indeed, these are simultaneous. Every clinical decision we take – about prescribing, about referring or not, about direction to other agencies – has a cost attached. Someone is paying that cost, either directly as part of NHS activity or indirectly through the costs of time off work and lost productivity. Our actions as doctors have major consequences for the UK economy. We need to become engaged in working out the extent and consequences of this.

The days of us saying 'we just practise medicine, it's too bad the system has run out of money' are coming to an end. We have enjoyed the idea of 'the purely clinical doctor' to whom the system will 'provide the medical profession with the best and most modern apparatus of medicine' for many years, but this has only been achievable within the protective cocoon of the large envelope of total NHS funds, and no one being held individually accountable. This stage of NHS clinical activity is coming to an end, and commissioning will force us all to become accountable both for our clinical activity and for making good use of the available funds. It marks a major challenge to our profession, a major (always present, but newly explicit) commission to our profession and a major opportunity for us to take. It creates many new highly skilled roles for us to fill, and it creates significant additional demand for sessional doctors. It also scares many doctors, in both primary and secondary care, and many doubt we are able to rise to this challenge and deliver.

IMPLICATIONS OF THIS

There is a need to match the activity of the medical system with the availability of resources, and as the main workers who commit NHS clinical activity and cost in certain directions and away from others, there is a need for us to look at what we are doing and see what we are achieving, and what we are failing to achieve. These things are clinically and economically necessary, and they will not happen unless somebody leads them – that is, someone taking the steps needed to get them to happen. They will not happen if we all keep going out of meetings to see another patient (rather like an empty in-tray, a patient-free time in medicine will never happen).

Variability among GPs is immense,[11] and shows up in differences in referral rates, prescribing costs and so on. As far as the system is concerned we may all be GPs providing a similar service to our list of patients. When viewed from an area-wide perspective it becomes apparent that some GPs provide the same service for far less total cost to the NHS system, and without obviously worse clinical outcomes. In other words, the variation in activity seems to be related to the doctor's behaviour, and not to demographics, economics or the prevalence and incidence of pathology. There is a phenomenon here to be explained, and we need to become part of that explanation and understanding. Sadly, our explanatory framework here has not caught up with our ability to describe the phenomenon.[12-14] At least as commissioners we are in a position to ensure clinical input into the development of this understanding.

So in general practice (and the other specialties of medicine), however much many GPs do not like to admit it, there is a need for the local medical system to be led, and for ordinary GPs to engage with the leadership processes. We are all parts of a whole bigger than ourselves. When we lift our perspective to this level then we start to acknowledge for a commissioning process and for this to be led. As GPs we, or at least some of us, will need to move beyond just seeing our work as seeing the patients and move to work on the wider system issues around our work. We will need to think about what we do as much as about the doing of it. And once we start thinking from this view then we have become system leaders as much as doctors.

GP CLINICAL COMMISSIONING GROUPS

I am a member of the nascent clinical commissioning group (CCG) in Calderdale. Along with nine other colleagues (from the 130 GPs in Calderdale) we are trying to work out our function, and turn ourselves into a decent commissioning organisation that brings our clinical knowledge together with that of the managers and their knowledge of activity and finance issues. So far we are working well together and are learning a lot from and about one another.

We meet each Thursday afternoon, sometimes as a group of clinicians and sometimes as part of the clinical commissioning executive at which we are part of the team that makes decisions about service changes and developments in Calderdale. We are privy to full financial information from the finance director. We see where and how the whole budget of NHS Calderdale is allocated. We are rapidly building strong relationships with council colleagues in the social care side and with our secondary care colleagues. We are building links with the voluntary sector. We think that our strength will be in our relationships and not in forcing more into and out of contracts.

We are about to take over many, but not all, of the functions of the primary care trust. Some of the primary care functions are being reserved to the newly forming National Commissioning Board. Some of the primary care trust functions are going to the cluster – the overarching group that brings NHS Calderdale (Halifax), Kirklees (Huddersfield) and Wakefield together. Some functions are best provided over a cluster area rather than by each individual organisation. There is still conversation going on about the exact final shape of the new structures.

Over time we think we have achieved a clinically focused, well-managed, collaborative way of working that will let us achieve better patient care for the patients in Calderdale. We think we can do this mostly via negotiation, relationships and persuasion. As far as we can, we want to avoid threats such as contract penalties.

THE FUTURE FOR CLINICAL COMMISSIONING GROUPS

The key question for me, for the commissioning group and for the NHS as a whole is whether the CCGs are the right vehicle for commissioning the whole NHS.

There is a tension between using the wide knowledge and experience of local GPs to drive improvements in the system with those same GPs also being providers within that system. There is a push in the NHS for more work to be moved into primary care. As GPs and GP commissioners, we clearly cannot act to direct NHS funds into our own practices. That would be utterly unethical and it would immediately bring charges of insider training and conflict of interest. However, if as commissioners we cannot direct activity towards primary care and other providers, we cannot innovate and move services closer to home.

The compromise at present is that the CCG can provide clinical advice to the cluster and the national commissioning board about what would be clinically useful in primary care in our area. The commissioning process, and money allocation, for any accepted proposals would then be run entirely separately from the CCG. This seems to get around the problem.

I think in time we will see some GPs move into commissioning work as a specialty in its own right, and work on developing pathways of care across primary, secondary and social care provision. I think other GPs will move into 'medical services provider companies' and specialise on the provision side of the system. For new GPs, there are opportunities here in both directions.

One current uncertainty about commissioning concerns how many functions will be provided by CCGs themselves and how many will be bought in from 'commissioning support organisations'. These organisations may be very helpful and take away some back office functions, thereby freeing up the time of CCGs for their main activity. If the commissioning support organisations act like this they will be helpful and useful. If they are an attempt by the centre to stifle CCG activity, innovation and discretion in decision-making then they will be resented, and they will hinder the whole process. Many people are worried that the commissioning support organisations will dominate the CCGs.[1,2]

So far the CCGs are developing well in many parts of the country, and the prospect of improved local and clinically informed decision-making seems within reach. The commissioning support units and the National Commissioning Board are not yet even operational. Remember that most of the things we worry about never actually happen; even if they do, we are resilient animals and we usually find a way of working around them.

THE RELATIONSHIP OF PRIMARY CARE AND SECONDARY CARE

NHS care provision is divided into primary and secondary care, along with bits of intermediate care and social care provided by local councils. The fundamental flaw of the NHS has been that it employs lots of intelligent people in such a way that they can only get in the way of one another. To some extent they can only do their job well by cutting across other people's paths.[9] The problem arises from silo-based thinking throughout the service. This silo-based thinking is buttressed by financial incentives that apply inconsistently across the service, so that what works for one part may work against the whole. Whether CCGs can end this silo thinking remains to be seen. There are endless boundary disputes, and if commissioning is seen simply as a process done onto secondary care by primary then the boundary disputes can only get worse.

Perhaps we should be looking to break down the barriers between primary and secondary care?

In the past, primary and secondary care have resembled nothing so much as an old married couple arguing over who gets more or less of a rather threadbare duvet. When they both realised that the duvet was empty they have held it out with loud wailing and demanded more filling. I believe in the DH this is called 'shroud waving'. As one of my Scottish patients reminded me, 'there's nae pockets in a shrood.'

The division between primary and secondary care in the UK is an accident of history that emerged between the Apothecaries Act of 1815 and the Medical Act of 1858. The division can be summarised as 'the GPs got the patient whilst the hospital got the diseases'. Iona Heath described this division and reviewed its effects beautifully in her Harveian ovation.[15]

There is a need to balance the work of primary care with secondary care and of system finance with clinical activity and the needs that have to be met. There is a need to direct the power of well-focused secondary care activity, with a filtering system that get patients who need it quickly to it, but which also keeps those who don't need it away from its risks. Barbara Starfield's work over many years showed how systems that had this balance worked better overall for patients.[16] The UK primary care system comes close to this balance,[17] and anything that damages the UK primary care system is likely to increase overall NHS costs and increase the population mortality.

Over time we will need to move towards thinking about systems and networks of care, with more local negotiation of pathways and clear allocation of responsibilities. We will be in conversation with secondary care and social care about where exactly the balance between us all should lie. In this way we will start to build a system so that even if a patient enters it at a wrong point they are quickly directed to the right point. The art of such design would be to arrange the nodes within it (e.g. surgeries, clinics, A&E departments, ambulances) so that they worked alongside one another, rather than as separate, free-standing entities.

It is going to be a major challenge for commissioners to achieve such harmonious networks, and it will involve much work by local GPs and consultants speaking to each other regularly, and by commissioners negotiating directly with the acute and mental health trusts. These conversations will be valuable, and certainly in Calderdale we are keen to encourage them and to develop them further.

The future ways of working in the NHS may look very different from our existing silos, and may well be all the better for the change. If we can lower the boundary between primary and secondary care and instead think of the system as experienced by the patient, and how they find their way around the well sign-posted network (as opposed to blundering through a partially charted labyrinth with care gaps to fall into and with large barricades between different service providers)[18] then we may be able to make the system work more sensibly for both patients and staff, and probably run more smoothly and cheaply. Remember that existing inefficient systems with many glitches run up all sorts of hidden costs: wasted time, staff ill health, stress, angst, aggravation, arguments, extra appointments, secretarial sorting time, extra faxing and so on.

To reduce this we need to be thinking at the level of whole pathways and systems of care and how we organise these well.

THE RELATIONSHIP OF CLINICAL COMMISSIONING GROUPS TO PRIMARY CARE

The CCGs stand in an odd relationship to primary care, being of it and yet not of it too. Some of the problems have already been mentioned here.

The CCGs are being asked to take a leadership role among their local member practices, and to lead the way in involving them in working on the system. For example, the CCGs are being asked to look at the variation in performance among practices and see how much is justified and how much needs improvement. This work will be approached collaboratively and initially in a frame of reference looking for understanding. There may be specific local differences between practices and areas.

Over time it is likely that practices and individual doctors will become more aware of how they compare against others in their area. This knowledge will of itself bring about some changes in behaviour – doctors are competitive, and do not like to be outliers on anything. If they are outlying, they are likely to want to think about what they are doing differently from colleagues, and to think of different ways they could direct activity. Elizabeth Evans *et al.*[19] have shown how such an approach based on education can lead to changes in clinical activity (not reducing referrals, but getting referrals refined and better directed – sensitivity the same, and specificity raised). Strangely the advice that 'more people need a good listening to than a good talking to' may prove very helpful to CCGs as they work with their constituent practices. Understanding may achieve more change than any guidance, instruction or sanction. In time, the practices and their CCGs will develop new ways of working together, and the process could be interesting and beneficial for both sides.

In 2007 the RCGP published a roadmap for the future of general practice.[20] In this document the authors saw that the current distribution of small practices was not sustainable for the future and that practices would need to become part of a bigger whole ('a federation') in time, and club together to provide more services collectively. Commissioning is one of the biggest opportunities we have had as GPs to make this happen. In terms of the roadmap it provides the forum, within which GPs can realise the vision:

> We urge that GPs organise themselves into a force to be reckoned within their local health economies. We hope that this document will be used by GPs and others as a basis for declaring an ambition to improve their local NHS.

SHOULD WE MOVE TO WHOLE-SYSTEM COMMISSIONING?

I think in time we will move to whole-system commissioning. We are already doing this as far as we can. There is a missing element in the debate and conversation when the primary care component is not involved in the discussions about the service – it is, after all, the key entry point for most care pathways.

A good recent example of this approach has been the improvement in management of acute cardiology services in England over the last 11 years, led by Sir Roger Boyle. What was once patchy and parochial has now become a coordinated regional network of collaborating services, hospitals and ambulances working to one goal of getting the cardiac patient rapidly diagnosed and receiving definitive treatment as quickly as possible.

If CCGs can mirror this success at their local levels they will achieve much. For me it is exciting to see this opportunity and to join in with trying to make something of it.

CONCLUSION

I hope in this chapter I have shown new GPs (and maybe some older ones too) some of the opportunities commissioning presents for GPs. To my way of thinking it presents the best opportunity for many years to get the conversation going across primary, secondary, mental health, social care and the voluntary sector, and to bring their work together so that the whole system works better for patients.

If we can achieve this we will have achieved much for the NHS. Far from it being the end of the NHS,[1] if we get this process right it will be the making of the NHS.

For new and old GPs alike, this set of changes creates many opportunities.

It is new skilled senior-level work for GPs, and it will increase the need for our skills, in commissioning, in filling the vacancies in the surgery, or in developing new provider services.

Leadership and followership are two important dynamics in anyone's career. It is well worth knowing how you relate to these concepts and what styles of leadership and followership you like and respect.

Commissioning is the latest attempt by the NHS to get its purchasing and service specification function right. It is a key new role for GPs (among others) and it is a major opportunity for our profession, which is why so many senior GPs are moving to take the opportunity it presents. For new GPs it may seem a bit distant immediately. At the very least it will create a need for more backfill to practices, and therefore more locum sessions.

What have you been commissioned to do as a doctor?

I now need to bring the discussion back to the level of a new GP. Think of your own career so far. What have you been commissioned to achieve as a doctor? What should you be working towards? Who are you leading already? Who will you be leading in the future? What qualities have you got? What qualities will you need to develop? Why will people want to be led by you in the future?

These are all questions around you, around how you see yourself as a doctor, and about how you see yourself developing through time. You may well be asked them at interviews. Your answers to them will change throughout your career as a GP. I'd encourage you to give a definite answer to them – the best you can give for now. At least you then have something to modify as you learn over time.

I hope you will enjoy considering them and answering them throughout and through the development of your career. The challenge I will always make to new GPs is to ask, 'Does your career go beyond your consulting room?' At some stage you will need to answer that.

REFERENCES

1 Gerada C. From patient advocate to gatekeeper: understanding the effects of the NHS reforms. *Br J Gen Pract*. 2011; **61**(592): 655–6.
2 Iacobucci G. RCGP and GPC call for 'super CCGs'. *Pulse*. 2011 Dec 14: 3.
3 DH 2011 NHS Operating Framework Available at: www.connectingforhealth. nhs.uk/systemsandservices/infogov/links/operatingframework2010-2011.pdf (accessed 17 December 2011).
4 Webster C. *The National Health Service: a political history*. Oxford: Oxford University Press; 2002.
5 Klein R. *The New Politics of the NHS*. 6th ed. Oxford: Radcliffe Publishing; 2006.
6 Haslam D. "Schools and hospitals" for "education and health". *BMJ*. 2003; **326**(7383): 234–5.

7 Department of Health. *NHS Atlas of Variation 2010*. London; 2010. Available at: www.rightcare.nhs.uk/index.php/nhs-atlas (accessed 17 December 2011).

8 Department of Health. *World Class Commissioning: vision*. London; 2007. Available at: www.dh.gov.uk/en/Publicationsandstatistics/Publications/PublicationsPolicy AndGuidance/DH_080956 (accessed 17 December 2011).

9 Davies P, Gubb J. *Putting Patients Last*. London: Civitas: Institute for the Study of Civil Society; 2009. Available at: www.civitas.org.uk/pdf/PuttingPatientsLast02July09. pdf (accessed 17 December 2011).

10 Garbutt G, Davies P. Should the practice of medicine be a deontological or utilitarian enterprise? *J Med Ethics*. 2011; **37**(5): 267–70.

11 King's Fund. *Improving the Quality of Care in General Practice: report of an independent inquiry commissioned by The King's Fund*. London: The King's Fund; 2011. Available at: www.kingsfund.org.uk/publications/gp_inquiry_report.html (accessed 17 December 2011).

12 O'Donnell CA. Variation in GP referral rates: what can we learn from the literature? *Fam Pract*. 2000; **17**(6): 462–71.

13 Davies P, Pool R, Smelt G. What do we actually know about the referral process? *Br J Gen Pract*. 2011; **61**(593): 752–3.

14 Wennberg J. Time to tackle unwarranted variations in practice. *BMJ*. 2011; **342**: d1513.

15 Heath I. *Divided We Fail: Harveian oration*. London: Royal College of Physicians; 2011. Available at: www.rcplondon.ac.uk/resources/harveian-oration-2011 (accessed 17 December 2011).

16 Starfield B, Shi L, Mackinko J. Contribution of primary care to health systems and health. *Milbank Q*. 2005; **83**(3): 457–502.

17 Commonwealth Fund 2010. *Commonwealth Fund Annual Report*. New York City; 2010. Available at: www.commonwealthfund.org/Annual-Reports/2010-Annual-Report.aspx (accessed 9 March 2012).

18 Lakhani M, Baker M. Good general practitioners will continue to be essential. *BMJ*. 2006; **332**(7532): 41–3.

19 Evans E, Aiking H, Edwards A. Reducing variation in general practitioner referral rates through clinical engagement and peer review of referrals: a service improvement project. *Qual Prim Care*. 2011; **19**(4): 263–72.

20 Royal College of General Practitioners. *The Future Direction of General Practice: a roadmap*. London: RCGP; 2007. Available at: www.rcgp.org.uk/pdf/CIRC_RCGP%20Roadmap%20Future%20General%20Practice%2013th%20Sept%202007.pdf (accessed 17 December 2011).

FURTHER READING

- Brereton L, Gubb J. *Refusing Treatment*. London: Civitas: Institute for the Study of Civil Society; 2010. Available at: www.civitas.org.uk/pdf/RefusingTreatment.pdf (accessed 17 December 2011).
- Gupta S. *Effective GP Commissioning – Essential Knowledge, Skills and Attitude: a practical guide*. Oxford: Radcliffe Publishing; 2011.
- Newdick C. *Who Should We Treat? Rights, Rationing and Resources in the NHS*. Oxford: Oxford University Press; 2005. A barrister's superb description of how processes are adjudged fair and unfair by the law. Essential reading for those interested in ethics and those involved in healthcare allocation decisions and the processes followed to make them – which is all of us.

ANALYTICAL TOOLS TO SUPPORT COMMISSIONERS

- Public Health Observatories (PHO), formerly Association of Public Health Observatories APHO general practice profiles (http://tinyurl.com/625czz2)
- Department of Health, Practice-based commissioning: budget guidance for 2011/12 – methodological changes and toolkit guide (http://tinyurl.com/64rp8g6)
- NHS atlas of variation in healthcare (http://tinyurl.com/6a4lbwb)
- NHS comparators (http://tinyurl.com/3vb9tcw)
- Office for National Statistics neighbourhood statistics (http://tinyurl.com/2cbufz)
- Primary Care Commissioning application (www.pcc.nhs.uk/pcca-application)
- Programme budgeting atlases (http://tinyurl.com/3t7zf8f)
- Programme budgeting benchmarking tool (http://tinyurl.com/67ldq5h)
- Spend and outcome tool (SPOT) (http://tinyurl.com/3mg2glf)

Chapter **10**

A day in the life of a GP

Peter Davies, Hussain Gandhi and Lindsay Moran

There is no such thing as a typical day in general practice. The day can vary tremendously depending on a number of factors such as whether you are a partner, a salaried or a locum GP; the support that you have in the GP practice (administration, nursing and GP support); whether you do on-call or out-of-hours work; and the demographics of the area you work in. This is not to mention other personal factors such as other job commitments and your general well-being and energy levels.

For those GPs working in low socioeconomic areas there can be a demand for urgent appointments, requiring a different appointment system from the book-in-advance one. There may be a demand for letters and social support. Equally, doctors working in high socioeconomic areas face a different type of demand: their patients can be highly educated and can attend with their internet printout in hand, detailing their condition and the treatment they wish you to prescribe. Working in areas with a high ratio of ethnic diversities can also bring challenges. Different cultures often have different expectations; for instance, they may want a GP to prescribe them antibiotics for their every ailment or they may simply want the GP to refer them to a specialist without further intervention in primary care. Alternatively, their expectations may be very low, meaning they will be very pleased with any small amount of care that you give to them. If there is a low prevalence of English-speaking patients then the use of interpreters brings its own time burden and challenges to the consultation.

In some practices you may find that you are the only GP working there; this is even more of a challenge to locum GPs who may not know the area, the staff or the patients. In any urgent situations that arise, you are the only person there to deal with the problems, no matter how many. If an urgent visit comes in at 5.55 p.m., then it's yours, irrespective of the pile of urgent paperwork on your desk, the patients awaiting your urgent phone call and the dinner you've planned later with your partner. At least in a practice with a number of GPs working, this burden is shared. This speaks equally true for the available nursing and administration staff.

There can be quite a difference between the workload of a new GP and a more senior GP. The senior GPs seem to handle so much more in comparison with new GPs. When viewed from the eyes of new GPs, senior colleagues effortlessly deal with difficult cases, calmly deal with what looks like a sinking ship and handle multiple tasks simultaneously, all without getting a hair out of place. The young GP, on the other hand, gets more and more stressed as they frantically scribble away at the ever-increasing pile of paperwork, dictating furiously and barking at patients when they step out of line, all the while with sweat pouring from their brow. As in all cases of experience, the more a GP does their job, the easier it becomes and the calmer and faster they become at getting the work done. Also, knowing your patients and not having to cross the bridge of rapport building makes handling cases easier and safer.

So, let's look at a couple of 'typical' days.

THE PARTNER GP'S TYPICAL DAY

There is no such thing as a typical partner day in general practice. The version presented here reflects my (Peter) work when I am in my surgery doing direct clinical work. I may think I am typical but others may think the same about themselves, and we are probably doing different things. Each surgery has a slightly different rhythm to its work.

0800–0830	Arrive at work, read any post, path links, say hello to everyone
0830–0845	3× 5-minute phone appointments with patients
0845–1130	16× face-to-face 10-minute appointments
1130–1200	Catch up on prescriptions, plan visits, handle any urgent requests
1200–1300	Visits (anywhere from one to seven, but usually two most days)
1300–1400	Lunch
1400–1500	Read daily post not read in the morning; write letters; work through list of insurance forms, reports, prescriptions, path links, emails, phone calls
1500–1515	3× 5-minute phone appointments
1515–1800	16× face-to-face appointments
1800	End of day (in practice I often leave the building at 1825).

That's the clinical specification, incorporating two clinical sessions in a day. It is very busy, and has a lot of activity within it, all done at a quick pace. But this day does not include practice meetings (Fridays, 1130–1300) or time for clinical audit, significant event audit, reflection, or commissioning work. It does not include practice development work. It does not cover QOF work. It does not cover various meetings with various people. All these activities are just fitted 'in and among', which explains why they are often missed out or not done well.

My practice has a duty doctor, so once my surgery is booked I am unlucky to get interruptions or any extras, except if someone is off work in an unplanned manner (e.g. a staff member has gone home sick). I am the duty doctor for emergencies each Wednesday. The surgeries are getting easier now that I have been in the practice 6 years and know most of the patients. I mostly run near time now, and the overrun is down to about 15–20 minutes.

Over the week I do seven clinical sessions as described in the table above. On Thursdays I have two sessions of clinical commissioning group work – for which I get paid separately.

My full-time partners do the above timetable for nine clinical sessions a week. They then say, 'we have no time to do anything else. Don't people know we are busy?' They are, but as always the question that someone like me will ask is, 'Is this really what you should be doing? Should you have a bit more variety within your work?' The choice, of course, is theirs to make.

THE FREELANCE GP'S TYPICAL DAY

It would be nice to state that as a freelance worker there is a particular structure to the day. However, one of the benefits (or disadvantages) of being a freelance GP is the variability. This too can vary tremendously depending on whether it is a short- or long-term post and whether or not you have agreed to do additional work for the practice beyond seeing patients.

A typical clinical day would follow a pattern similar to that of the partner GP.

0800–0830	Arrive early, orient myself with the practice and systems in place, say hello to everyone (remember to make sure you can log on to the computer)
0830–1100	15× face-to-face 10-minute appointments (number of appointments and duration can vary pending negotiation with the practice, but this is the average)
1100–1200	Catch up on the sorting out of paperwork from the clinic, network with staff, plan getting to visits (if agreed)
1200–1430	Visits, lunch, networking, self-directed learning, personal time (varies pending work agreement)

1430–1700	15× face-to-face appointments (again, varies pending negotiation with the practice)
1700–1730	Ensure all paperwork is done
1730	End of day (I leave on time).

This may seem a more appealing day than a partner's day. However, it does represent a difference in roles between the two, a difference in responsibility and, as shown, a variation based on your agreement with the practice. One major variation that can occur is working at two separate practices on the same day, which will add in time pressure to ensure punctuality.

A non-clinical day can vary from personal time, including holidays, to self-directed learning, courses, working in other roles (i.e. teaching, appraisal, other occupation roles, leadership, commissioning), or more personal aims such as writing, exercise or self-development. The variety is the attraction. The ability to be comfortable with long-term variety is a key factor that determines how long a person works as a freelance GP. Again, the choice is each person's to make.

THE SALARIED GP'S TYPICAL DAY

A typical salaried day often mirrors that of the partner GP's day already described or, in some jobs, the freelance GP's day. The salaried GP usually gets involved in the paperwork, signing prescriptions, reviewing the path links and being included in meetings. It is usually everything as already described but without getting involved in the running of the business. A salaried GP is often there to do more of the clinical work, releasing the partners' time to allow them to give more to the running of the business. Salaried GPs may take on more of the business roles if perhaps they are looking to take on a partnership role in the future. So, the role of the salaried GP can vary a lot depending on what their contract is with the practice.

Whatever your role is in general practice there is no doubt it will be fast paced, full and never dull.

Chapter 11

The doctor's bag

Hussain Gandhi with input from Lindsay Moran

The doctor's bag – a time-old, classic piece of equipment that, being carried by you as you march down the street to the aid of a patient, announces to the general public who you are. Traditionally the doctor's bag was made of brown leather and was self-standing and top opening with a split handle. Big enough to carry all the necessary equipment but small enough to be portable, today the doctor's bag has diversified into something that can simply be functional, something that provides safety and something that allows you prestige, style and class. It can portray who you are and make you look the part. Many high-end brands have their own versions of the doctor's bag now – Biba, Whistles, Chloé, Chanel, Gucci, Louis Vuitton, Ralph Lauren and Coach, to name but a few – and you can expect to pay anything from a few hundred to a few thousand pounds for these. Alternatively, if you are not into the bling and the brands, there are many high-street shops now marketing versions of the doctor's bag, or you can even improvise with a smart computer case. A metal tool case from B&Q is an excellent alternative – good for compartments and even better for sitting on during those home visits where there is no suitable seating available for whatever reason!

There are various suggestions regarding what should be in a doctor's bag. The following lists of items are meant as a brief guide.

ESSENTIAL ITEMS
- Bag – it's a good idea to have a lockable bag, especially if carrying drugs and/or patient-identifiable information items
- Stethoscope
- Diagnostic set (otoscope and ophthalmoscope with a blue filter)
- Thermometer
- Sphygmomanometer (manual or electronic)

- Torch (especially useful for home visits in winter)
- Sample pots/swabs – you will regret not having them when you need them
- List of local hospital numbers
- *British National Formulary* or equivalent
- Urgent medications: aspirin, glyceryl trinitrate spray, salbutamol inhaler, spacer and so forth; if unable to gain from practice, use private script and keep the receipt
- Conversion chart of opiates and palliative care medications (easily obtainable from local hospice or palliative care nurse)
- Examining kit: gloves, lubricating gel, hand-cleaning gel and clean wipes
- Stationery, spare pen, paper (headed, if need be), FP10 prescription form.

OPTIONAL ITEMS

- Pulse oximeter
- Glucose monitor and strips
- Extra-large cuff for sphygmomanometer
- Tape measure
- Peak flow meter and spare tubes
- Urine MultiStix
- Benzyl penicillin (this can be considered essential, but it is important to note expiry dates)
- Rectal diazepam
- Injectable medications (i.e. analgesia, anti-emetic, adrenaline and so forth)
- Tendon hammer
- Phlebotomy equipment with sharps bin
- Tongue depressors
- Fluorescein dye
- Basic first aid equipment, plasters, bandages and a rescue mask (for mouth-to-mouth resuscitation).

NON-BAG EQUIPMENT

Some items are not specifically part of the 'doctor's bag' but they are still important to carry. These include:

- photographic ID
- phone/smartphone
- local map or satnav
- warm jacket and/or wellies
- snack and water bottle (for those really busy days when you do not have time to go find one – very valuable if working as a freelance).

NOTES TO CONSIDER

Being a mobile doctor carries with it a few legal implications to bear in mind.

- **Insurance**: both for transport (i.e. car) and for your bag. Check the terms of your policy to make sure you are covered for business use; this can be a costly mistake if made and you need to make a claim. You may need to insure your bag separately.
- **Controlled drugs**: you are able to carry controlled drugs; however, it is important to note the regulations in doing so and to keep appropriate records and disposal methods.
- **Information governance**: if carrying patient notes and so forth for visits, remember there are various rules regarding storage and governance; do read your local guidelines but do not carry such information unless necessary, and never leave this information unattended in your car or on display.

APPLICATIONS

As well as your doctor's bag and all the items in it, most doctors now carry around smartphones or notebooks to make their working life easier. I (Hussain) maintain that such equipment will become as essential to a GP as a stethoscope in the impending future. Alternatively, there are computer programmes or websites to turn to for help with clinical practice. The world of technology is having a profound effect on the way we deliver healthcare. One of the most recent changes has been the shift from software to applications or 'apps'.

The following are some useful apps that can be used in your day-to-day working life:

- **Evernote**: a great free notepad app that can be used as a stopgap to your appraisal and revalidation ePortfolio. Great for taking notes, photos and videos to link to your continuing professional development work, Evernote is available on most platforms. If you need higher storage limits these can be obtained for a fee.
- **MIMS**: although the British National Formulary app is more well known, the MIMMs app is of equal quality and provides equal depth of information as far as drug guidance apps go, and at nearly a fifth of the cost. This is available on Android and iOS.
- **VisualDX**: a great dermatology app that can be used for comparing rashes, or even as a differential diagnosis aid. It is reasonably expensive, although this is less than the cost of a dermatology course. This is available on Android and iOS.
- **Epocrates**: a combination of MIMS with a medical calculator. This is free to use though a large download and available on most platforms.
- **Google Translate**: not as good as a translator, but it does come close and

it is very useful if Language Line is not an option. This is available on Android and iOS and through any internet browser.

- **PocketCPR**: a cardiopulmonary resuscitation guidance app offering real-time feedback and an audible metronome. This is available on Android and iOS.
- **Google Navigation**: if you have an Android phone please download this app. It is a satnav for your phone and it runs off Google Maps. This app makes finding your way to home visits a doddle.
- **MedCalc**: a collection of medical calculator programmes in one app. This is available in iOS.
- **3D Brain**: as it sounds, this is a great app to help understand neurology. This is available on iOS.
- **Pillboxie**: if your patient has an iPhone, get them to use this app. It helps them to effortlessly remember when to take medications and, more important, it shows them which one to take. This is available on iOS.
- **NHS Direct**: the NHS has their own app for information for patients. This is a basic but useful app that gives medical advice.

Chapter 12

How to stay sane and healthy as a GP

Peter Davies

Show me a sane man and I will cure him for you.

—CG Jung

The patient is the one with the disease.

—The Fat Man, from *The House of God*

WHY DOES A DOCTOR'S HEALTH MATTER?

Doctors are an unusual group of patients. We know a lot, but we are far from good at applying our knowledge to ourselves. We deal with patients well and mostly find it a straightforward process. It is what we are trained to do. When it comes to applying our knowledge to our own symptoms we are rarely accurate, and yet we are often reluctant to ask one of our colleagues to apply his or her well-trained medical gaze over us. It is often difficult as a caregiver, to then become the receiver of care. As the old saying has it, 'a doctor who treats himself has a fool for a patient'.

In some ways doctors can be seen as a group whose health needs are poorly catered for. We care for others, but the provision for us is limited. Other groups of senior professionals such as company directors, senior lawyers and managers have their health screening sessions at BUPA Wellness or the Nuffield, or similar. I used to think these medicals were a waste of time, and medically their value is dubious, in terms of revealing pathology. Having done some work on them in the past (it's enjoyable and fairly paid), I think I now realise why companies ask for them and regard them as a fairly priced maintenance cost for hard-working, stressed, senior staff who are an expensive asset to maintain. The companies who pay for these medicals are not very interested in the senior partner's hernia or earwax or their slightly raised cholesterol. What they are keen to see is who has got stressed beyond reason, who is drinking too much, who is struggling to stay fit enough to keep up with the demanding work roles. They are a gentle way of discovering such matters and getting medical and other help in place earlier rather than later, and before the senior partner drinks away all the profits and loses all the clients. Sadly, there is no similar system in place for senior NHS doctors, although with higher rates of alcoholism and suicide than in the general population, there probably should be.

The key point about a doctor's health is that there is the risk of a double tragedy. The sick doctor needs care and attention just like any other patient. The risk of a sick doctor is to their patients. If a doctor's illness leads to impaired performance at work, then rather than having a single tragedy we may get multiple tragedies: **a sick doctor, impaired work performance, harmed patients and professional disciplinary processes activated against the doctor.**

ILLNESS AND THE GENERAL MEDICAL COUNCIL

Illness may be little or no defence against disciplinary charges – the harm has happened to the patient and has to be acted upon. However, the GMC does have procedures in place to take health factors into account, and it modifies its case handling accordingly. In appraisal each year we are asked to make a health declaration. This may seem fussy and routine but to the GMC the old scenario of a doctor's illness not becoming apparent until the performance issue arises is no longer acceptable. The key issue for the GMC is that a doctor who has a problem is honest about it and seeks clinical and if necessary occupational health advice and treatment for it. Such a doctor shows insight, and the fact they had had their illness treated would confirm this. The doctor who could end up in problems at the GMC is the one who has signed off all the health declarations as 'no problems' and then when a case comes in tries to claim illness as exculpation. Such a doctor has either put his or her own health at risk and not got it treated or has a dangerous lack of insight into the risk his or her illness poses to others. **Denial and lack of insight are danger signs to those investigating medical performance issues**. The health issues that most commonly catch doctors out here are drug or alcohol addiction, or severe depression.

(A brief note is needed here to remind readers that the illnesses that affect doctors most commonly are coughs, colds and backache – just as for the general British population. These illnesses however are treatable, and are relatively minor and with little risk to anyone else.)

The serious mental health conditions such as severe depression and addictions are all conditions often hidden for many years by their sufferers. As a doctor if you have one of these you are far better to get it treated than try to hide it, both for your own health and for your ability to continue in the profession.

As a doctor, I need to make sure that I am sane and healthy both for my own personal flourishing and so that I can treat the patients well. When the GMC guidance starts with, 'You must make care of the patient your first concern', there is a hidden presupposition here that the doctor is well enough to actually do this. If as a doctor you are not well enough to do this, then you need to get treatment for your own sake and for that of your patients.

The health of doctors is an issue in patient safety, and this takes concerns about our health way beyond our individual problems and concerns. We have a public persona as well as our private one. We do matter significantly to many, many others.

THE STRESSES OF MEDICINE

The stresses of medicine are many. All doctors are to some extent wounded by their experiences as doctors. We all have seen sad cases, badly managed cases and difficult cases, and we have dealt with traumatic experiences. We have probably all had periods of 'relationship dysfunction' and 'poor communications' with colleagues. We will all have endured a few rows and arguments. We may have had to handle complaints against us that, no matter how baseless, still tax our patience and coping abilities. We are supposed to keep a calm, amiable and equable disposition while all around us, and maybe inside us, is a mess of seething, emotionally charged events, reactions and responses.

Now all this is of course a part of medicine, and we have to learn how to handle it, and to be 'professional' and 'detached' and 'not to get caught up in the emotions of the situation'. However, we also need to accept that medicine does make significant emotional as well as time and technical demands on its members. Yes, in the heat of medical action we have to focus on the task at hand and do the job. We cannot allow ourselves to become paralysed by emotions – we have to remain able to think and act. But every so often we need to step back and reflect on how we handle the load of sadness, grief and stress that we encounter in our work. We are not without emotions. We are passionate and compassionate people, and our work is never 'merely technical'. Medicine done well is never 'just business'. Our work matters to patients and our pride in doing it well is the strongest defence against bad medicine. Doing your job well is one of the strongest ways known of boosting your own health and self-esteem.

Therefore, as doctors we need to acknowledge the stresses of our job, and we need to put in place strategies that will allow us to deal well with these stresses and without harm to ourselves, our families, our colleagues or our next patient. Also, as colleagues, we need to avoid harming one another too. 'First do no harm' applies to colleagues as much as it does to patients.

Illness in a doctor is a personal problem for the doctor concerned, just as illness of any sort is for the patient affected. The risk of a doctor's ill health is both to the doctor as patient and to the doctor's patients. **The key point about our health as doctors is to not let our ill health become a problem for others as well. As in first aid, we need to avoid the second casualty.**

Tragically, in the past many doctors have struggled on at work with severe illness as they will say they are 'unable to take time off' and 'wouldn't dare to let my colleagues down' or 'show any weakness'. Many doctors still see illness as a personal failing in themselves and others, rather than as a problem to be dealt with. This is harsh on ourselves and, indeed, daft – most of us are actually very good at dealing with problems, once we have diagnosed them.

When we are dealing with members of the public as patients we are professional and kind, and if they want some time away from work we usually give it to them. When we are dealing with ill colleagues we sometimes act almost as if we have forgotten how to be compassionate to each other. The patient is the one with the illness and you're a doctor, not a patient. It is almost as if we cannot, or will not, cope well with the concept of 'doctor as patient', either for ourselves or in our colleagues. Sadly, if you are ill as a doctor you may find that your colleagues are not as supportive as you would like, unless you have a disastrous major pathology.

Some colleagues take a great pride in their 'presenteeism'. They are never ill, and they have never had a day off sick in their lives. They sound like the old middle-aged Yorkshire business owners who'd say, 'I've never had a day off sick in my – [collapses]'. General John Sedgwick's classic, 'They couldn't hit an elephant at this dist –' comes to mind, and we do well to retain a bit of humility in the face of the many forces of pathogenesis.

Now, the scenario I have described is readily recognisable to all of us, but the fact is that most of us do not crumple under its demands, and most of us do not succumb to stress. Most of us show **resilience** in our personal and professional lives. Even when we have setbacks, mostly we recover from them. We call this recovery 'experience', and even though it may be bitter, what does not kill us makes us stronger. It can be seen as being like a psychological version of the immune response.

> All of us know that we are as vulnerable to pathology as any of our patients. Indeed, we know our vulnerabilities more – what else is medical knowledge but the catalogue of the ways in which mind and body can go bad, mad and sad? What else is life but a highly prevalent, 100% fatal, sexually transmitted illness? Like the orthopaedic surgeon's view of athletes, we come in three types: those about to get ill, those who are ill already and those recovering from illness. We know all too well how dust crumples into dust, and ashes into ashes.

HANDLING STRESS

They say that stress is the tension experienced between knowing that the unreasonable person you are dealing with really needs a good thumping and knowing that you are not allowed to deliver this much-needed corrective.

Sometimes it's an inchoate rage, and you don't know who or what deserves the good kicking, but you are damn well going to find out and administer it. People help you in your enquiries, and eventually the wiser people around you point out that it is 'Roger' who (fortunately) is away for 2 weeks on holiday. You save your anger up for his return, but by then it has dissipated, and you move into problem-solving mode. You smile when you see him and say, 'Hello Roger. Welcome back. There was a little problem while you were away, but it's sorted now.'

Hans Selye, who defined the term stress and described the autonomic responses that go with it, now admits that he used the wrong engineering metaphor. He feels he should have used the term 'strain'. Stress is the feeling we get when we are under physical and/or mental strain.

The experience of stress is subjective: what is stressful for you may be of no concern to me. Likewise, you may wonder why I have got so stressed when the incident seems so minor to you. Stress is an **outcome from an event**, and **our internal physiological and mental responses** to that event. The events in life and work are not going to stop anytime soon, so we really have to learn to deal with how we respond to events, and with how we assign meaning to them. Bear in mind that the brain may respond and assign meanings to events very quickly, and turning these reactions into considered responses may take some time. Knowing a way of hiding your immediate reactions is a useful skill in medicine. In medicine we often have to experience the stress, and then deal with it later.

My colleague Dr Seth Jenkinson introduced me to a useful 'problem-solving fork'. He said that any problem can be sorted in one of four ways:
1. denial
2. sorting the problem
3. sorting out how you respond to the problem
4. moving away from the problem.

Denial is effective for a short while, at the expense of much mental effort, and sometimes absurdity when the denial becomes unsustainable. It is very commonly used, especially by government departments as a first step in trying to deflect attention away from a problem, on grounds that if everyone stops talking about it then it is no longer happening. Watching denial collapse into absurdity is either good fun or horrifically fascinating, depending on where you are observing from.

Sorting the problem is obviously the best answer, but often times you are not working at a level, or with enough position or persuasion power, to do much about it. For example, many significant event systems ask what steps the reporter has taken to prevent a recurrence. The steps needed are often not those that an individual can take, and the specific individual incident report needs considering in the context of other signals received from multiple sources across an area. The remedial action needs taking at a level above the one at which the problem is experienced. Often you just do not have the personal resources or authority to directly solve a problem.

So you then have to work on **sorting out how you respond to the problem**, and how you go about defining it, and working with others to sort it, and how you avoid getting frustrated with it. As a general rule, the key difference here is between a disorganised mess of misunderstood facts, high emotions and lack of organisation and a problem that emerges when you get clarity of definition and a focus on a solution, to at least part of the mess. There are whole fields that help people with this adjustment, and cognitive behavioural therapy, psychology, neurolinguistic programming and many other techniques all have some successes in helping others with this. Ultimately they all reach a point where you 'get your head around it'.

Moving away is sometimes a valid problem-solving option. Certain scenarios are basically insoluble, and dangerous. The classic example here is the battered wife who goes into a women's refuge for her own safety. There may be good reasons in certain scenarios to move away from a problem quickly. However, many people are too quick to use this option when, with persistence, a problem may eventually become soluble. Others, however, are too stubborn and they leave moving on too late, getting bogged down with a problem for too long, to their own frustration, and blocking the way for someone else to tackle it. Hitting the golden mean between these extremes is far from easy, and sometimes others may spot your predicament before you recognise or still later acknowledge it. Very smart people know when to move on and call it 'career development'.

I could say much more about this topic, but it is better at this point to direct you to the further reading suggested at the end of this chapter and let you find your way to learning your own strategies about how to handle stress. You probably have many good ones already.

TYPES OF STRESS

Medicine is intrinsically stressful. Every day you either see stressed patients or you are stressed yourself, or both. It pays all of us to learn about coping with stress, both for ourselves and for our patients. It is worth looking at the types of stresses we face in our work. Some stress we have to accept as part of our work. A difficult operation, an acutely ill child, seeing patients you are fond of die, breaking bad news and so on are all intrinsically stressful events that are a routine part of medicine. However, it is to be hoped that as your training has gone on you have learned to deal with such events, such that although they are stressful, you will feel that you know what to do to handle them reasonably well. And you realise that sometimes the outcome will be bad, no matter how well you act. A cardiology registrar once said to me about heart failure patients, 'Yes, they do die, don't they?' It was just what I need to hear, and it allowed me to treat my heart failure patients more sensibly, with recognition that their prognosis was limited, and that I could not stop all their deaths, and that I would not be blamed for their deaths.

The intrinsic stresses of medicine are something that we need to accept. However, much of our stress arises from other sources. Some of our stress is **internally generated**. Doctors (and lawyers, and many other professionals and skilled workers) tend to be perfectionists. We want to make everything right. We want to do it in the right way, and yet we work under time and resource constraints that hinder our efforts at every turn. We can easily get frustrated that 'everything is (conspiring) against us' and 'how am I supposed to do good work when this system is so awful?'

Perfectionists make great doctors – they are conscientious and hard-working – but they can easily become stressed and highly strung, and this may tip over into depression. They work to high standards, but at a personal cost. **The frustrated perfectionist** is a common archetype in medicine, and if you see one provoked, it's best to move out of their way until their anger has calmed. Ward sisters used to be superb at turning up with a cup of tea in their office at just the right time to calm many a frustrated perfectionist down. GP receptionists are often good at this too. (Remember to say thank you to them after they have bailed you out.)

A lot of our stress is **externally generated**. They say the NHS used to be 'doctor centred', but if you call the mishmash of misaligned activities and incentives you can observe any day in a surgery 'doctor centred' then I wish to dispute with you. The NHS is often an inefficient monocultural monolith that sometimes runs like a tank with unoiled wheels. It sometimes steers like one too. There are a lot of frustrations and silliness in how the systems are set up to run. Why do midwives fax results to GPs rather than just issue a script themselves? Why have we not authorised and trained them to use a list of basic medicines as routine training? Why can a senior nurse not give paracetamol to a patient, while in the next bed a clueless 16-year-old has administered 100 tablets to herself? Why is a nurse who can give intravenous drugs at one hospital in town not allowed to give them in the other hospital in town? Does her brain become mush as she crosses from one side to the other? Why can an item be prescribed by a GP but not by the hospital consultant? Why do doctors have to prescribe dressings and food supplements they have barely heard of rather than get the district nurses or dieticians to prescribe in their own right?

There are many, many examples of silly and frustrating systems in the NHS. Why they have not been solved years ago, I do not know. My mother (a 77-year-old retired eye surgeon) listens to me for a while and then replies 'Your father [a consultant eye surgeon from 1968 to 1990 – he died in 1999] had that problem too.' Yes, the late discharge summary and stray letter are the hardy perennials of the problem weeds in the NHS garden. All NHS enquiries conclude, with all the great wisdom that can only arise from profound hindsight and regret that 'communication needs to be improved'. You would have more fun starting from the universal answer and asking, 'Now, what's the question?'

Sometimes the world is mad, and the madness is to tolerate it. I am one of George Bernard Shaw's unreasonable men who won't. ('The reasonable man adapts himself to the world; the unreasonable one persists in trying to adapt the world to himself. Therefore, all progress depends on the unreasonable man.'[1])

Perhaps 'being reasonable' should be seen as a form of madness?

GENERATING HEALTH AS A DOCTOR

We have talked enough about stress in medicine. I now want to talk about how we can maintain our health and sanity as doctors. The job is as it is, and like all jobs it has its stresses, strain and madness. I doubt that as doctors we are worse frustrated perfectionists than those in other professions such as law and accountancy.

Despite the stresses of our work, most doctors are reasonably happy, and reasonably healthy. Although we have some risks to our health, we are well paid, highly intelligent professionals who have far more control over our lives than most of our fellow countrymen. Our overall mortality rates are low compared with many other professions and with lower social classes.

So how do we maintain and generate health as doctors? As I described in my paper 'Between health and illness',[2] we need to remember that **health is the constantly evolving outcome from a life lived well**.

How we feel on any given day is a balance between the processes of salutogenesis (health generation) and pathogenesis (disease generation). The balance between these processes is mediated by homeostasis.

In this section I want to look at what helps generate health for us. **Wealth** is the first thing to mention. Wealth and health derive from similar roots. As the study of health inequalities shows, the richer you are the healthier you are and the longer you live. There's a strong correlation between education and wealth generating ability. So **being well educated** gets you good jobs that generate wealth, and tend to leave you healthier. As a doctor, you start from here.

Second, **respect and esteem** generate health. We are social animals and we cannot live fully free of the good or bad opinions of others. As doctors we get a lot of recognition from our colleagues and our patients. Getting additional qualifications such as a master's degree or your college fellowship are good esteem boosts.

Third, **physical fitness** is helpful – fitter people think more clearly and withstand stress better. Their cardiovascular system is stronger.

Fourth, **resilience** is the antidote to stress. We look a lot at stress, but most of us do not buckle under it. Human beings are resilient, and able to withstand many stresses successfully.

Fifth, **relationships** are helpful. You can never be too good at relating to your family, your children and your colleagues – and, one would hope, a few friends from other activities. Relationships with friends generate health. Appropriate use of **mood alteration strategies** is useful. These can all be underdone or overdone, but if they are done to the right amount they can be helpful.

- Advisable – sex, exercise, religious activities, group activities, alcohol, coffee, chocolate, salt, food, antidepressants, thrill seeking (e.g. rock climbing), relaxation, writing, hobbies.
- Inadvisable – illegal drugs, drunkenness, crime, fights, smoking, too much of the advisable activities, overtraining, driving too fast, installing wife 2.0 and hoping wife 1.0 won't mind, having an affair with the practice nurse.

Sixth, a **sense of coherence** – a sense that things make sense, that we have a place and a role in the world and that we can make some difference by our actions. This leads on to a sense of **personal effectiveness**.

Seventh, a **sense of humour** is useful. In medicine we see a lot of **the absurd**; we see many versions of Sisyphus pushing heavy burdens uphill only for those same burdens to flatten Sisyphus as they roll back downhill. We know that all efforts are ultimately futile. Somewhere along the way we must find a source of **meaning and purpose for our lives**, either a religious system or, as Sartre described for the atheists, we must make our own version.

Eighth, **being involved** is important. The elements already mentioned combine to leave you in a healthy place from which it becomes natural to be involved in whatever activity you choose. The activity is likely to have purpose, and to lead to many other relationships, that make life interesting and allow you to learn much more from others. Sartre said that 'hell is other people'. We need to remember that so too is heaven. My basic belief is that the more interesting people I can meet, the more fun I will have and the more learning I will enjoy.

So we can see the elements we need to have in place that should help us stay sane, healthy and resilient. Finally, remember the Oslerian wisdom of 'Normal? Normal? What do you mean normal? The only person who's fully normal is the one we haven't examined properly'. Marry that up with Jung's insight: 'Show me a sane man and I will cure him for you'. We are none of us entirely normal, and we all have our oddities.

As someone has suggested, 'an eccentric has learned to be happy with their neuroses, while the neurotic is still unhappy with their eccentricities'.

To your good health.

REFERENCES

1 Shaw B, *Maxims for Revolutionists*. Project Gutenberg; 1903.
2 Davies P. Between health and illness. *Perspect Biol Med*. 2007; **50**(3): 444–52.

FURTHER READING

- Bennet G. *The Wound and the Doctor: healing, technology and power in modern medicine*. London: Secker & Warburg; 1987.
- Ghodse H, Mann S, Johnson P, editors. *Doctors and their Health*. Sutton, Surrey: Reed Business Information; 2000.
- Rowe L and Kidd M. *First Do No Harm: being a resilient doctor in the 21st century*. 1st ed. Sydney: McGraw-Hill Medical; 2009.
- Siebert A. *The Resiliency Advantage: master change, thrive under pressure, and bounce back from setbacks*. Illustrated ed. San Francisco, CA: Berrett-Koehler; 2005.

Chapter 13

Dealing with isolation and medical uncertainty

Peter Davies

Managing uncertainty is a major part of medicine. It is something we do every day, whatever specialty or niche we are practising in. We are all making decisions on partial information, on probabilities rather than certainties. We are all doing this quickly, and of course we are all making some mistakes as we do so.

One of the major changes a new GP will realise immediately is that they are now outside the safety of the vocational training scheme and a training practice. There is not a trainer ready to debrief you after a surgery. There is not a course organiser to ask (although most course organisers will help young GPs who ask them for it).

Anyway, you are now the doctor, and the patient is entirely your responsibility. You are in a new surgery and you do not know which of the partners to ask. You do not want to look incompetent so maybe you are afraid to ask. The patient is in front of you expecting answers. And now you find yourself not sure about what to do. You need your strategies for managing uncertainty to work.

WHAT STRATEGIES MIGHT HELP HERE?

First, make sure you have **a good history** – more uncertainty is resolved by a good history than anything else.

Second, make a decent assessment of illness severity. What is your immediate impression as to whether the patient is *well* or *ill*? This first impression judgement is surprisingly accurate; good doctors, and often casualty sisters and paramedics, are very good at it. If you train yourself to make this judgement well, then your medical life becomes easier. It is usually comfortable to work alongside a confident health professional who can make this judgement call well. Working alongside someone who cannot make this call well is difficult.

You will rarely go wrong to check pulse, temperature and blood pressure, peak flows, oxygen saturations and urinalysis (according to the clinical scenario), even if only to give yourself a bit of thinking time. If they are all normal the patient is unlikely to be immediately ill, and even if they become ill later at least you have examined them properly. Many patients have suffered harm from delayed diagnosis, poor recognition of disease severity, and under-treatment of their condition for lack of simple measurements being made. For example, if you read any of the confidential enquiries into asthma deaths the theme of failure to perform a peak flow test, and therefore failure to realise the severity of the asthma, is a contributing factor in many of these deaths.

Try to get the timescale of the illness right. Is it acute? Is it acute on chronic? Is it chronic? Generally, the faster the onset of an illness then the faster it needs to be dealt with. How fast do myocardial infarctions, sub arachnoid haemorrhages or strokes need to be treated? How long can a blood pressure check wait? You will realise that acute severe life-threatening illnesses tend to have short definite histories. Conversely, if the history meanders over the patient's dietary and bowel habits over the last 20 years then there is unlikely any major or new pathology present or undiscovered. Think of such histories as story time rather than medicine time.

Is there a condition present with a risk of rapid deterioration overnight? If so, does the patient know what to do if that happens? Or would you be better to admit him or her to forestall any problems? As one of my GP trainers, Dr Cliff Godley, explained to me, '**if you are going home worrying about such possibilities you should probably have admitted the patient**'. These days GPs are coming under increasing pressure not to admit patients and instead to try to handle problems in other ways. However, if the other ways are not obvious, or if they are not easily available, and the doctor has a worry about the patient that cannot be managed at home or in primary care, then the GP has to do what is right for the patient and decide to make the admission. Sometimes it takes courage to do this despite the critics – you need to be decisive and courageous – and inquests and the General Medical Council are more frightening than a few muttering consultants, commissioning group members and managers. All those people who talk about 'alternative pathways of care' are not there in your evening surgery, and they will not rush to defend you in the coroner's court or General Medical Council if there is any comeback against you. (If commissioning works well then there should overall be fewer occasions in which the scenario described arises, as the alternative pathways will have been activated ahead of time, anticipating the need. For the time being, such scenarios are very recognisable to any practising GP and the alternative routes are still under construction.)

Consultants on acute units may mutter about 'too many inappropriate admissions', but when they are more reflective they accept that their judgement is retrospective, and made with the help of time, and rapid access to detailed investigations that can rule serious pathology in or out quickly. The GP does not have this speed of access to tests, and if there is a risk of a serious pathology it is safer to **be oversensitive** (detect most cases, but also admit some that come back clear of pathology) rather than **overspecific** (be right, but at the risk of missing cases). At the end of the day, the risk is to the patient's safety and well-being. Have you minimised this risk by your actions? Or have you taken a risk where the patient will bear the potentially serious downside consequence?

Then, is this a new or repeated problem? One of the easiest and most effective rules in medicine is that if the patient has had it before and thinks it is the same thing again, then it probably (>90%) is the same again.

On a related theme is the GP 'rule of threes'. This states that the first time a symptom is presented, you can do anything. The second time you have to get it right. If it presents for a third time then it is probably time to ask for outside help such as a referral. This rule applies whether the problem is seen by the same doctor or by three colleagues across a practice, or among a GP, and out-of-hours service and an A&E department. Once a symptom has been presented at the surgery three times, then the solution is probably going to come from beyond the surgery.

So we have here the basics of assessment of acute illness, and I hope what I have written above is a reminder of things you know rather than being new to you. It will mean more to you as a young GP now that you are implementing these decisions for yourself.

Acute severe illness you need to recognise and deal with. If what you are dealing with is acute and severe then you need to treat it as such, and in general practice **recognition of severity** is as important as an **exact diagnosis**. The example of meningitis illustrates this well. For example, I once went to see a sick baby at its home on a Sunday morning. I picked up the family's concerns rather more than any obvious examination findings in the baby. I admitted on the basis that the family were usually sensible, and therefore probably right to be concerned. The diagnosis came back as pneumococcal meningitis, and the child was treated successfully.

WHAT ARE THE OTHER PROBLEMS THAT GENERATE ANXIETY AND UNCERTAINTY?

I suspect other scenarios generate much uncertainty, probably needlessly. Once you have excluded acute severe pathology you should find yourself with time to think through and consider the scenario. You may now have time to arrange a second consultation and a later review. Maybe some bloods or X-rays in the meantime would help? Or they would at least exclude some easy-to-spot conditions and allow you to cover QOF bloods as well for the year. As long as you are confident that you are not missing acute severe illness, or a subacute possible cancer, then you can give yourself time for an illness to emerge or resolve.

I suspect that for many younger GPs the conditions that cause them most problems are those that are not serious but which are **miserable morbidity**, and which lead to repeated visits to the surgery. For example, what exactly is a good treatment of plantar fasciitis? Were you asleep in that bit of the medical course? Have you read that bit of the textbook? Having seen a case, will you now turn it into a doctor's educational need and look the condition up? There are lots of these minor but annoying conditions that you will rarely see in hospitals and which you will not see very often in practice. However, over time you will see most of them a few times, and you will become like a classic general physician who has seen or read about a case of every disease.

For all of us, garnering this knowledge and experience takes time, and it involves seeing enough patients with enough different pathologies to get to know them. For young GPs in a rush this will be annoying, but, **ultimately, persistent disciplined practice** is what distinguishes the expert from the non-expert in anything. Geoff Colvin describes this beautifully in his book *Talent is Overrated: what* really *separates world-class performers from everybody else.*[1]

Skin rashes baffle the best of us, even dermatologists, often. They are often worth a second opinion from a colleague. Usually this is as much to rule out pathology as it is to make a definite diagnosis. Skin rashes that are recognisable (e.g. acne, psoriasis, shingles) are usually easy. The more difficult cases are ill-defined rashes with no obvious precipitant and no obvious diagnostic label to apply. Sometimes 'Betnovate-sensitive erythema' is as good as we can achieve. In my own experience, when I was a young GP on the out-of-hours service in East Kilbride, a colleague, Dr Shakeel Ahmed, twice helped me diagnose erythema multiforme. He'd read that bit of the dermatology textbook. I had too, but I had not really understood it. I was glad I had asked his help, and we learned from the conversation. I still missed it a third time, and a paediatrician gently corrected me. I have diagnosed one or two successfully on my own since then.

Getting an internal second opinion on many problems is useful. Doctors mostly enjoy discussing cases, and swapping ideas with one another. As a young GP you may be pleasantly surprised by how much your more experienced colleagues enjoy discussions with you – either regarding pathology or regaling you with stories about how to manage a certain family. You may be surprised to realise how often older GPs have forgotten things and find it useful to plunder a newer doctor's brain for ideas about a case of their own. The more colleagues you can meet and greet and learn from the better for you, and for them. How I am as a doctor now is the result of my meeting and learning from many patients and colleagues over the last 28 years. Thank you to all of them.

Your general pathology knowledge is often very helpful. It often allows you to specify a process in play in a clinical situation. For example, you may not have the name of the illness but if you can identify inflammation and infection you have a therapeutic approach to the problem. Identifying the pathological processes in play is often a very useful strategy for navigating uncertainty.

Conversely, identifying what is not in play can be positive, in that you can give the patient specific reassurance. For example, 'no, it is not chickenpox.' Sometimes being told 'this is not a case of x' is what the patient wants and needs. It is nicer when you can get to a defined diagnosis, but sometimes putting the important negatives in place is the best we can do.

Acknowledging ignorance can be a useful strategy. Who among us does know everything? Patients are often not fooled when we bluff them, and they may well respond positively to 'I don't know what is going on here . . . but I will find out . . . by means of . . .' The key point for patients is that at least their problem has been heard and that some attempt is being made to define it accurately.

Phoning a friend works well and in the medical context your friends include primary and secondary care colleagues. Often a phone discussion will help you resolve your uncertainty, and although consultants are busy (as are you) they mostly enjoy discussing cases and deciding if they need to be in their clinic or not. Some versions of Choose and Book software now have an advice option that can be used prior to launching a full referral. Consultants often find GPs difficult to get hold of. If you have left a message for a consultant to ring you back and you are then going to be away on some other activity, you would do well to give both the surgery number and your mobile number for the consultant to call you on.

Sometimes the best answer to a situation is 'as much nothing as possible'. The situation may be indefinable or intractable and insoluble. Any attempt to make it better is then liable to make it worse. For example, some people's depression is existential: like Eeyore, they will always find another thistle to munch on, and they may even enjoy telling you ('that nice young doctor who listens to me so well'). I had one of these once as a young GP dealing with a lonely older woman. I made all sorts of helpful suggestions to her, all straight from the geriatric medicine textbook. She managed to turn down every one of them for some reason or other. Eventually I worked out it was just how she was, and she had set her life strategies to make her lonely many years before I got to meet her. For all she was presenting at the surgery she didn't seem to want much to do with our treatment suggestions. Voltaire once stated that 'medicine is the art of keeping the patient entertained whilst nature cures the disease'. Sometimes our job is to keep the patient entertained. Alternative medicine providers are often very good at this, and if there is no major illness present, they are often helpful in this task, having more time and more entertaining explanations than we manage.

Finally in this section, **remember that management of uncertainty is the art of general practice, and no one has fully got it right**. Even experienced GPs are still struggling with it. It is to be hoped that you will get better at it over time, but you are unlikely ever to totally master it. Anyone who is ever totally happy with their management of uncertainty is probably too complacent. The next section explains why.

SYMPTOM SOUP

Biomedicine occurs at the intersection of the iceberg of disease with the iceberg of symptoms. In a GP setting the incidence of symptoms is far greater than that of pathology. Many, maybe most, symptoms have little or no pathological significance. Many diseases have no specific symptoms. These considerations lead to major intellectual and practical problems with the classification of diseases, and the attribution of symptoms; the phenomenon of a drowning doctor clutching at diagnostic labels is well recognised. Erythema rubifaciens anyone? Idiopathic, of course.

The problem for both doctors (whatever age and experience) and patients is that we are trained to think that all symptoms are due to anatomical or physiological (including mental) dysfunction; a symptom suggests pathology and therefore a need for explanation and investigation. My old trainer Dr Douglas Murphy likened an experienced GP to a pike watching many fish go by before deciding to pounce on the one that really was a tasty morsel. Others describe GPs as managing '**symptom soup**'. I was discussing this one time with Professor Martin Roland and he pointed out that symptom soup is a bit like minestrone: mostly thin gruel, but with some significant morsels of pathology floating around in it.

Sadly there is very little guidance available on how to manage symptom soup. For some reason experts seem to like producing guidelines on specific, defined, already diagnosed conditions rather than on managing the range of ill-defined symptoms present in an average consultation. There is much guidance on 'how to manage a myocardial infarction'. There is much less on how to manage musculoskeletal or non-cardiac chest pain in the community. When assessing symptoms in the GP consulting room the approach taken by Hopcroft and Forte in their book *Symptom Sorter*[4] is extremely helpful – it's like the *British National Formulary* for medical problem-solving.

Watching GPs in action over time shows us that there are two extremes in our strategies for dealing with symptom soup. At one end of the spectrum are **oversensitive doctors** – those who react to many symptoms and may therefore end up diagnosing, treating and referring more often. They are therapeutically active and tend to end up more popular, as patients know these doctors will take their symptoms seriously and do something about them. Younger GPs are more likely to be towards this end of the spectrum.

At the other end of the spectrum are **overspecific doctors** – those who do not like to make diagnoses until they are clear. They investigate rarely and selectively, with high specificity, but they may have relatively low sensitivity. They refer late, if at all, and often the patients go on to other doctors who will refer them. To many patients, such doctors may seem aloof or uninterested. Their more activist colleagues may describe them as showing a lamentable lack of curiosity. Over time, as experience and knowledge grow, GPs tend to move more towards this end of the spectrum, especially as they come to realise that not every symptom necessarily needs to lead to a diagnosis.

Somewhere between these extremes is a golden mean of sufficient curiosity, adequate investigation and sensible referral making. Finding this golden mean is difficult; it the art of sensible general practice. The position of the mean alters over time, depending on whether low referrals and good gatekeeping are what is wanted, or whether we are being criticised (e.g. by the cancer tsar) for investigating too little and referring too few patients to the hospital. GPs can always be criticised for over- or under-referring. We cannot ever get it totally right. We need to be phlegmatic and sensible and work with colleagues to patiently get it more nearly right each year.

For practical purposes, knowing where you are on the spectrum between medical hyperactivity and a lamentable lack of curiosity and care is useful. If you want to measure your position on this you need personal referral and prescribing data over many years. In analysing such data we tend to assume that the data is normally distributed, and that those in the middle of the distribution are about right. However, this may be an example of fools seldom differing rather than of great clinical acumen or organisational insight.

Young GPs tend to be relatively high referrers. They have less experience both of medical conditions and of the patients in a particular practice. They may also spot more new pathology, which the older partners may have overlooked. Sometimes fresh eyes are very useful in a practice at the clinical level, as well as at organisational levels. Patients often take advantage of the opportunity for a review by a new doctor. Have the confidence to make a referral if that is what you believe the patient needs to help their care. You may be wrong, but on the whole I would prefer a doctor who asks questions more often than less. So too would most consultants. In many ways, in terms of detecting pathology, the GP's job is sensitivity (finding all the cases) and the consultant's job is specificity (sorting out the cases). **Don't be too worried if you are oversensitive. Do what is right for the patient at the time**, while accepting that with hindsight the decision may later appear wrong. The retrospectoscope is the only 100% sensitive and specific medical instrument and it only ever gives one report which is, 'told you so'.

WH Auden captures this idea beautifully in his poem 'If I could tell you':

> Time will say nothing but I told you so,
> Time only knows the price we have to pay;
> If I could tell you I would let you know.[5]

In general, doctors are fast learners – given what we need to know, we need to be! The more time you spend practising medicine the better you will become at recognising signs and symptoms and dealing with illness and medical presentations. Malcolm Gladwell, echoing the work of Geoff Colvin and many others, writes that the key to success in any given field is to clock up a total of 10 000 hours of disciplined practice doing that specific task. A new GP working eight sessions a week will take an average of 11–12 years to reach this golden number. At that time, you might want to sit back, put your feet up and feel smug that you are now a master at your art. Fortunately, life and events will happen to remind you not to be so careless.

SUMMARY

As a young GP you may be struggling with the management of uncertainty. It is difficult and there is a knack to doing it well that takes time to learn – this knack is what defines a good GP. The management of uncertainty is one of the perennial themes of general practice, and experienced GPs find it difficult too. The techniques in this chapter should at least keep you and your patients mostly safe – it is better to err on the side of caution. Do what is right by the patient, not for the commissioning budget or the area's mutterers.

REFERENCES

1 Colvin G. *Talent is Overrated: what* really *separates world-class performers from everybody else.* London: Nicholas Brearley; 2008.
2 Syed M. *Bounce: the myth of talent and the power of practice.* London: Fourth Estate; 2010.
3 Gladwell M. *Outliers: the story of success.* London: Allen Lane; 2008.
4 Hopcroft K, Forte V. *Symptom Sorter.* 4th ed. Oxford: Radcliffe Publishing; 2010.
5 Auden WH. *Selected Poems.* New York: Vintage; 1979.

Chapter 14

Adapting consultation skills to the world of actual general practice

Peter Davies

In your GP training you will have learned a lot about the consultation and about how you personally do it and how you should do it. Everything you have learned about communication is useful and, indeed, valuable. Briefly, you can never be too good at communicating. Communication skills are useful for medical practice for three powerful reasons, two of them positive and one negative.

- First, the negative: bad consultation skills place you at a higher risk of complaints and General Medical Council problems. You'd be keen to avoid these, wouldn't you?
- Then the positives: if you communicate well with patients, then you actually get to know them as people, and you begin to like them and enjoy your meetings with them. You may as well treat people you like – it is much more fun treating people you like than enduring people you do not like!
- Even better, if you communicate well with patients they will actually tell you what's wrong with them, so you get your diagnoses and problem definition more accurate, which is both good for the patient and more satisfying for you as a doctor.

However, there is a major gap between the consultations skills you learn on the vocational training scheme and demonstrate for the MRCGP exam and what can be achieved in the confines of a series of 10-minute consultations, plus interruptions, plus extras, plus other distractions that go into making up the average surgery of a British general practitioner.

Put simply, British general practice is run against the clock, and as a service it tries to do too much too quickly. Some things just have to give. Many years ago

Sir Clifford Allbutt characterised general practice as the 'perfunctory work . . . of perfunctory men'. These days we should acknowledge the force of his barb, and of course add 'and women'. To a large extent the confines around our work mean that our work can only ever be perfunctory. We are working at a systematic disadvantage that is prevalent and intrinsic to the structure and financing of our work. The new General Medical Services contract from 2004 has simply enshrined this systematic flaw, and missed an opportunity for a step change in general practice quality. As John Glasspool and I wrote in the *BMJ* in 2003,[1] in an editorial arguing for voting against the new contract:

> Where was the intellectual overview, the setting out of assumptions, the map to the future in any of the contracts? What were the contracts trying to achieve, and what reasons did they give for wanting to achieve these things? These are big questions about purpose that we now need to ask ourselves, whether as doctors, patients, or managers. As Kierkegaard says: 'Whoever has a why to live will find a how to live'.
>
> Specifying work patterns, blood pressure targets, immunisation targets, and such like are the details in all this, not the purpose of the contract. Irritation over too many patients and endless extras are details that inevitably emerge from the current system because we have not mapped out what we should be doing and what we should not be doing.

In short, the structures and processes in UK general practice are not currently set up to enable the achievement of the best outcomes for either patients or doctors. I have described this as 'the crowded consultation'.[2] They are a hindrance to good practice, and in time (I'd do it now, if I got the chance) they will need radical revision. I would argue that the structures and processes in UK general practice need to be altered to give the GP time and space necessary to get their primary function right. I see the GP's primary function as being that of accurate problem definition – in terms of a deep understanding about what is bothering the patient, and what pathology is likely to be present. If this primary problem definition is accurate, then subsequent decisions such as prescriptions, investigations and referrals are likely to be accurate and therefore also better targeted and more effective. They will also ultimately be cheaper, as the right patients get referred and the others are redirected away from the high costs of additional medical care. The recent papers from The King's Fund[3] and the Health Foundation/RCGP commission on generalism[4] argue along similar lines to this.

Anyway, the new General Medical Services contract has come in with all its many flaws. To be fair, it at least saved partnership general practice from imminent collapse at the time of its inception. However, it missed so many opportunities to improve the quality of the care that GPs are able to provide. It entrenched the incentives running in every GP surgery and through every GP consultation that value speed and access over quality, safety and thoroughness.

Your GP training will have mostly focused on the individual consultation[5-7] and the individual clinical problem. In practice you will be dealing with a surgery full of 15–20 consultations, each of which may cover many clinical and administrative problems. The pace of your problem-solving will have to increase rapidly, and this is one of the major stressors in the early years of general practice.

If it is any consolation, it remains one of the stressors for experienced GPs. General practice surgeries are fast paced and stressful. It takes a lot of skill to successfully bring a surgery to a conclusion at the right time, with the major pathology picked up and the minor worries allayed successfully. You can never get too good at this. As you get to know your patients more it gets easier, but there are two dangers here: time brings complacency and a lamentable lack of curiosity. A new or younger doctor may well come in and with fresh eyes notice something that has passed unnoticed by the more experienced colleague. Do what is right for the patient, even if the senior partner will be embarrassed. Ultimately, your partners will respect you for doing what is right for the patients.

The trick here is to do this in such a way that you get the medicine right for the patient, without implying that the other doctor has forgotten his medicine. A quiet conversation will often be useful. Beware you may spot what your seniors have missed, but they may be sharp themselves and spot a few things you've missed.

I have a great regret that having spent much time and effort during my training and afterwards on learning all these great consultation skills, the prevailing system in UK general practice stops me from using these skills fully. I expressed some of this frustration in my article 'The beleaguered consultation', published in 2006.[9] In that article I identified 13 threats to the consultation that threaten the effectiveness of the process. These threats are:

 1. time scarcity
 2. resource scarcity
 3. fear of our own inadequacy
 4. loss of tolerance and trust
 5. misuse of medicine to illegitimate ends
 6. indecisive management
 7. passive and active aggression
 8. complaints
 9. excess of expectations
10. litigation
11. loss of continuity

12. loss of confidentiality
13. media misrepresentation.

All of these are still in play, and as a fully qualified GP you will need to know how to deal with them.

If I wrote that article now I would see the consultation as more resilient than I then gave it credit for, with slightly greater tolerances. I do not think this is because of great medicine but, rather, that this largely arises because of the intrinsic tolerance and low expectations of the British population, the ability of the negligence lawyers to miss many open goals, and the lack of a readily available comparison and alternative to the NHS.

UNLEARNING SOME CONSULTATION SKILLS

On the vocational training scheme you learn great consultation skills and how to use them to open up discussion. As an experienced GP you learn when to open things up, and when there is a can of worms that you would rather not open, particularly in the last consultation of the night, when you are tired and thinking of home.

I am aware of how much I have come to use techniques such as ignoring minimal cues, or deliberately not asking certain questions of certain people on certain days. I am aware of how often I use differential reinforcement to direct consultations. I am aware of how much I steer consultations, hopefully safely and sensibly, but sometimes I just need to get back into medical harbour and I do not always give my best to every patient. All GPs do this, but only a few of us are honest enough to admit it.

In each surgery we all do many things – connections, referrals, prescriptions, listening – but any conscientious GP will be aware of how much more could be done, if we had more time and resource. As the writer Thomas Hardy put it, 'The petty done, the undone vast.'

This phenomenon of course explains the academic game of pronouncing that 'GPs are ideally placed to recognise this condition' and then in the follow-up paper, 'but sadly GPs seem to miss this condition on many occasions'. Well, of course we do. We each do much in our surgery, but there is much that goes undone, unsaid and unrecorded (and unappreciated, unrecognised and unpaid).

Dr Linus Geisler, a German professor of medicine, has written a useful communication book[10] that he begins not with a preface but with an apology to patients. I quote it here, and can only admit that I have done all these things often, in self-protection, from fear, in a rush:

- I have spoken rather than *listened*.
- I have been given *wrong* answers because I have not asked the right questions.

- I have misunderstood my patients because I have *not recognized* or have *confused* the various messages that they have sent to me.
- I have remained 'professional' rather than bringing empathy into the situation.
- I have *rejected* patients rather than *accepting* them.
- Discussions with my patients used to be unsatisfactory for both parties, because there was no *correct beginning*, no *clear definition of objectives* and no *concrete conclusion*.
- I have generated *time pressure* and made it obvious that I was rushed.
- I have *ordered* rather than *motivated*.
- I have treated patients as if they were '*difficult*'.
- I have overlooked *anxieties*, and created them during discussions.
- I have not understood that *reality* for the patient was *not identical* to that which I believed to be true.
- I was not aware that *speech* is the most useful instrument that a doctor possesses.

> Briefly: I acted as do many of my colleagues. In doing this, I have missed many opportunities, disappointed hopes and have cheated myself out of part of the fruits of my work. I am now aware that the right dialogue between doctor and patient can bring about almost anything, but that incorrect dialogue achieves almost nothing. This book is a personal attempt to demonstrate the correct way in which discussions between doctor and patient should be carried out.

If you have not yet demonstrated all these flaws I have little doubt that soon you will be doing so – sadly, time constraints in practice make this inevitable.

There is a knack to knowing how to end a consultation, ranging from subtle (a glance at your watch, fidgeting, speeding up motor tics) to blatant (looking out of the window, staring at your watch, washing your hands for a long while, opening the consulting room door as the patient says, 'and . . .'). There is a time and place for all these strategies to get through overloaded, overpacked, overrunning British GP surgeries. If a patient is reading this and recognises that I have used one of these tactics on them, I can only apologise and hope that I made up for it at a later time, on a better day.

Other hints I can offer for dealing with overcrowded consultations include the following.

- Flushing out the agenda at the start. 'What have you come to see me about today?' Followed up with, 'and after that, is there anything else? . . . and anything else?' Keep going until all items are listed, and then see if it is realistic to tackle all the items in one 10-minute consultation or if some will have to be deferred until another appointment.

- Some patients have unrealistic expectations about how much can be done sensibly in one consultation. They may have 'saved it all for today' to try to make things easier, but this is rarely helpful to their doctor. If you cannot deal with all the agenda in one consultation then it is perfectly fair to prioritise and insist that some of it is deferred to a later consultation.
- One consultation is for one patient – and no, you cannot see three children as well as the mother.
- Summarise accurately and ruthlessly; if your summary is wrong, revise it.
- Your guess as to what type of person someone is is likely to be accurate. This may be stereotyping, but most doctors are good at this. It is sensible to check if you are right, but if you confirm your suspicion you can then often use past knowledge of similar types of people to help produce an answer quickly and accurately. A version of 'my friend John' or 'other people I have seen who were in a similar position to you' may then let you introduce a solution to them. Of course we are all unique, just like everyone else.
- Remember that GPs are (or should be) good at both recognising patterns of people and patterns of diseases.
- The pattern of attendance over time is a physical sign in its own right – look at past attendances and their patterns.
- Always look beyond the confines of the current consultation. The current consultation is often merely an event thrown up by underlying biological, psychological or social processes, and this event may or may not be amenable to treatment. The content of the consultation means little if not understood in its context.
- In medicine, past performance is usually a very good predictor of future performance.
- Sometimes your best ability is to do 'as much nothing as possible'.
- Sometimes you just need to listen harder. As Dr Chris Manning puts it, 'Don't just do something, sit there!'

I have a feeling that the quick, brief consultations in British primary care actually are counterproductive, in that they fail to allow us to properly define the problem, either in terms of the patient's concerns or in terms of likely pathology. This failure of primary problem definition leads to mistakes and also to unnecessary activity such as extra referrals and investigations, as it is easier to arrange these than it is to find the time to think clearly and really define the problem. Simon Cocksedge has written a useful book titled *Listening as Work in Primary Care*.[11] Sadly, all too often listening is not seen or valued as work in general practice – it is too slow and it is not efficient. Surely you should speed up and run to time more often? This pressure to run to time may actually be the most time-consuming and resource-wasting step in the whole NHS.

At the practice level it leads to repeated appointments until eventually one of the doctors actually gets a grip on the problem. The feeling of what Balint called 'collusion of anonymity' is large.[12] In this phenomenon the patient and the problem are passed among multiple doctors and specialists but no one ever really accepts the responsibility for dealing with it. In today's medical system of micro-specialisation the potential for this is growing with each referral, resulting in a letter back that goes, 'not in my area of specialism' rather than giving a positive steer to the patient's journey.

Once you are beyond your vocational training scheme (and maybe during it) some consultations will take you to the 'edge of chaos'.[8] Learning to live on this edge is both exciting and terrifying; as an experienced GP, I quite enjoy taking patients to this edge, but I know how to bring them back as well. Some of the best insights for patients come when you take them to the edge of chaos, and such consultations test the nerve of even experienced GPs. You will learn a lot if you learn how to navigate this edge well. Many colleagues both young and old avoid it and so miss the chance to really develop their ability. They become like cricketers who only ever score singles, never hitting a four or a six.

In summary, you will adapt your consultation style with experience. A good history is still the basis of any good medicine. And medicine is much more enjoyable when you can do this well, both because you enjoy meeting the patients more and because you get your medicine done better. Good consulting is one of the joys of general practice. If I show my frustrations with it is because I feel that it happens despite rather than because of the system we work within. Good consultation is the basis of good medicine, and should happen by default, because the system makes it easy to deliver. Sadly, in the NHS it happens at personal cost to the doctor, in the stress and difficulty experienced in trying to get each surgery done well and completed on time. Many doctors manage one or other of these but few get the balance between speed and accuracy absolutely right.

Finally, remember the opening statement of this chapter: Communication skills are useful for medical practice for three powerful reasons, two of them positive and one negative.

- First, the negative: bad consultation skills place you at a higher risk of complaints and General Medical Council problems. You'd be keen to avoid these, wouldn't you?
- Then the positives: if you communicate well with patients, then you actually get to know them as people, and you begin to like them and enjoy your meetings with them. You may as well treat people you like – it is much more fun treating people you like than enduring people you do not like!
- Even better, if you communicate well with patients they will actually tell

you what's wrong with them, so you get your diagnoses and problem definition more accurate, which is both good for the patient and more satisfying for you as a doctor.

Good communication keeps you out of trouble and lets you score highly on both the *scientia* and *caritas* parts of your work. This is a pretty good payback for a few smiles and using a little intelligence deciding when to talk and when to shut up.

REFERENCES

1 Davies P, Glasspool J. Patients and the new contracts. *BMJ*. 2003; **326**(7399): 1099.
2 Davies P. The crowded consultation. *Br J Gen Pract*. In press.
3 King's Fund. *Improving the Quality of Care in General Practice: report of an independent inquiry commissioned by The King's Fund*. London; 2011. Available at: www. kingsfund.org.uk/publications/gp_inquiry_report.html (accessed 17 December 2011).
4 Health Foundation. *Guiding Patients through Complexity: modern medical generalism*. London: Health Foundation; 2011. Available at: www.health.org.uk/ publications/generalism-report (accessed 17 December 2011).
5 Neighbour R. *The Inner Consultation: how to develop an effective and intuitive consulting style*. Lancaster: MTP; 1987.
6 Willis J. *Friends in Low Places*. Oxford: Radcliffe Medical Press; 2001.
7 Dowrick C. *Beyond Depression*. Oxford: Oxford University Press; 2004.
8 Innes AD, Campion PD, Griffiths FE. Complex consultations and the 'edge of chaos'. *Br J Gen Pract*. 2005; **55**(510): 47–52.
9 Davies P. The beleaguered consultation. *Br J Gen Pract*. 2006; **56**(524): 226–9.
10 Geisler L. Doctor and patient: a partnership through dialogue: new ways of mutual understanding. Frankfurt am Main: Pharma Verlag; 1991. Available online at: www. linus-geisler.de/dp/dp01_introduction.html (accessed 9 March 2012).
11 Cocksedge S. *Listening as Work in Primary Care*. Oxford: Radcliffe Publishing; 2005.
12 Balint M. *The Doctor, His Patient and the Illness*. 2nd revised ed, 2000. Edinburgh: Churchill Livingstone; 1957.

Chapter 15

The business of general practice

Adrian Roebuck

This chapter will particularly interest you if you want to become a GP partner. However, as the provision of general practice changes within the NHS, having a sound and balanced awareness of the running of the business has never been more appropriate to all GPs, whether a partner or not.

This chapter is designed to provide some insight into the business aspects of general practice and to whet your appetite for spending time with business managers and practice managers to develop your knowledge and understanding of this key area.

While we often think of general practice simply as a provider of healthcare, it is much more than this. Indeed, behind this external perception we know that many practices across the UK are multilayered businesses – businesses that need to be well managed and efficient if they are to survive against the increasing demands placed upon them.

In the UK, general practice is run on a small business model. As a salaried GP, a successful business will ensure your continued employment and present and future career opportunities. As a partner, you are self-employed and with this comes great responsibility. The success of your business determines the costs that you are liable for and, ultimately, the profit you make.

SURELY IT'S ALL ABOUT THE PATIENT, NOT THE MONEY?

The funds available to the NHS and, indeed, to each general practice are finite and the patient still remains at the heart of what we do. The challenge in the current climate is to ensure we operate as efficiently as possible so that we do not waste money and we get the best possible care for every pound spent in pursuing improved patient care . . . this has never been more true.

Even the most optimistic individual can see that the costs within general practice are rising while income is at best static. In fact, in recent years, many general practices have seen a marked decrease in income and one can only imagine the pressure that is felt in those businesses as they try to balance the competing demands of increasing patient needs and the increasing costs of providing these.

Many people talk about healthcare demand in the UK being insatiable, as the population becomes both more needy and more aware of treatments and support available via the NHS. In addition, as we embark on our journey with clinical commissioning groups and the changes within the NHS we will see a greater need to effectively meet this increasing demand while managing the financial aspects of the provision of these services – no easy task!

PROFIT IS SECONDARY!

GP partners are remunerated through what is often called a 'drawing' – essentially this is their share of anticipated profits that the business will deliver. At the end of each financial year, the profits are calculated by the practice's retained accountant and any difference between actual and anticipated profit will need to be dealt with. If there is a surplus, the partners may wish to keep this money in the business until a later date or they may wish to take it as an extra drawing. If there is a deficit then the partner(s) may need to take immediate action such as injecting sufficient capital into the business. This is never an easy decision and with good advice from their accountants, such actions should have been anticipated and proactive measures taken, i.e. a planned reduction in drawings relative to the recalculated profit levels for the year.

As you can see, any cost pressures and resultant impact on profits will be felt most by the partners. Despite this, we should not just focus on the profit. Remember, profit is an output of all that has been achieved (or not) and it cannot be the only consideration for a business. **Profit itself is a very simple thing – it is the result of income less the costs incurred in achieving that income.**

CASH FLOW

It is a fact that a large number of failed businesses do not close their doors because they are not profitable but, rather, because they simply run out of cash! Cash is the lifeblood of any business and I would go as far as saying that cash flow is king!

Many businesses are financed through external investors who provide loans, mortgages, leases and so forth, and when these organisations 'feel the squeeze' they will often 'call in' their debts. If a business doesn't have the spare cash to repay this debt or if it is not able to refinance with another provider then it will often have to sell its assets or, indeed, use all its working capital to finance this repayment. This often means that it cannot continue, as it has no monies available to purchase products or services and so it ultimately ceases trading.

Therefore, the first step is to recognise that if we are indeed a business then we must manage our costs, drive our income and, importantly, plan for the future.

Many factors affect cash flow within a GP practice. The payment structure of the NHS is a key driver, with all its complexities (and often slow payment!). Most practices are paid their basic income from the NHS on a quarterly basis *in advance*. This is a great help with cash flow, but it requires good financial awareness and planning to prevent this money being spent early and there being nothing left in the latter weeks of the quarter to pay any liabilities!

However, as in many businesses, we are very susceptible to late payments from companies. One quick example relates to GP registrars who will be paid at the end of the month for their work in the practice and the associated claim for this that is not reimbursed to the practice until the middle of the following month. This may seem like small change, but a practice with a couple of GP registrars will need to allow around £12 000 of cash flow to bridge that gap between paying out the monies and receiving the associated reimbursements.

I'm sure your practice manager will also be able to tell you about creditors who have not paid their bills for months or, unbelievably, sometimes a year or more – over all of this time this is money that you cannot use in the business.

TERMINOLOGY

At this point it would be worth explaining some of the terminology used within the business field of general practice. There are various types of practice contracts:

- **General medical services (GMS)** – the term used to describe the medical services provided by a GP practice, who, in effect, are private businesses who are contracted to provide primary care on behalf of the NHS. This is the most established contract within primary care and latterly has been superseded by two new contracts which have sought to develop the terms between the provider (PCT) and the performer.
- **Personal medical services (PMS)** – here the practice and the PCT enter a local contract. The PMS contract pays GPs on the basis of meeting set quality standards and the particular needs of their local population. This approach has brought a wide range of benefits, being used to develop new services for specific populations, to attract doctors and nurses and to improve services for patients.
- **Alternative provider medical services (APMS)** – a contractual route through which PCTs can contract with a wide range of providers to deliver services tailored to local needs. It was introduced to allow PCTs to make arrangements outside of the established contracting routes with additional providers. Under APMS, PCTs are able to contract for primary medical

services with commercial providers, voluntary sector providers, mutual sector providers, social enterprises, public service bodies, GMS and PMS practices (through a separate APMS contract) and NHS trusts and NHS foundation trusts.

There are also some pertinent finance terms that would be useful to know:

- **Global sum** is a payment made to a practice that is determined by the size of the practice's patient list, adjusted for age and gender of the patients (children, women and the elderly have higher weights than young men because they cause a greater workload). Also, the practice gets an adjustment for rurality (greater rurality causes greater expenses), morbidity and for the cost of employing staff (the 'market forces factor', which captures differences in pay rates between areas, i.e. it is more expensive to hire a nurse in London than in Bradford).
- **Notional rent** is a reimbursement of rent by the PCT to the practice for allowing their premises to be used for NHS purposes. The PCT will establish the current market rent or the actual rent of the premises if it is a leased building, whichever is less, and review this value on a 3-yearly basis.
- **Direct enhanced services** are special services or activities provided by GP practices that have been negotiated nationally. Practices can choose whether or not to provide these services.
- **Local enhanced services** are special services or activities provided by GP practices that have been negotiated locally with the PCT based on local healthcare needs. Practices can choose whether or not to provide these services.
- **Minimum practice income guarantee** is used to top up practices' global sum payments – to ensure the practice receives an income at least equal to the income received before the new GMS contract. The payments made under minimum practice income guarantee are called correction factor payments. These are being phased out in favour of an increase in the value of QOF (*see* next point).
- **Quality and Outcomes Framework (QOF)** – described as a voluntary incentive scheme for GP practices in the UK, rewarding them for how well they care for patients. The QOF contains groups of indicators, against which practices score points according to their level of achievement. The QOF gives an indication of the overall achievement of a practice through a points system. Practices aim to deliver high quality care across a range of areas, for which they score points. Put simply, the higher the score, the higher the financial reward for the practice. The final payment is adjusted to take account of the practice list size and prevalence. The results are published annually.

- **Quality, Innovation, Productivity and Prevention** – a programme that is all about ensuring that each pound spent is used to bring maximum benefit and quality of care to patients. The NHS needs to achieve up to £20 billion of efficiency savings by 2015 through a focus on quality, innovation, productivity and prevention. Every saving made will be reinvested in patient care by supporting front-line staff, funding innovative treatments and giving patients more choice.

INCOME STREAMS

Fundamentally there are two income streams within a GP practice at the highest level: **core NHS income** and **enhanced income**.

Core NHS income is the funding provided against the practice contract (i.e. PMS, APMS, GMS) to provide 'core' primary care in your locality. As mentioned, this is paid to the practice each quarter in advance. Without getting engrossed in how funding is calculated, core NHS income is built around the size of the practice's patient list. The monies within the contract are for the practice to provide core services (both acute and preventive) to these patients, as required.

As we know, socio-demographic factors play a large part in determining the general health and well-being of individuals. At practice level this translates into increased or decreased demand and use of the services that a GP will offer. As such, the funding also takes into account the socio-demographic status of the population – four major factors being (1) gender, (2) age, (3) ethnicity, and (4) wealth, with many other measures also contributing.

Practices are very limited in where they locate their premises, as they have to be in the locality of the population they serve; therefore, the core contract will also pay the practice the relevant cost of being located in the area. These costs include actual/notional rents, business rates and water rates, but they do not include other items such as gas, electricity or telephone.

Within the core contract all primary care providers are rewarded for their achievement of high standards of care – better known as QOF. You may hear some people discuss QOF as though it is a bonus to practices for delivering against set targets. There will always be a healthy debate around this, but QOF can also be viewed as money that is within the core contract that can be retained (i.e. not paid if standards do not meet set criteria). QOF currently has 1000 points available in any given financial year; the value of each point will vary from practice to practice (again partly due to the patient mix we looked at earlier) but can be worth as much as £250 per point – that is a total value of a quarter of a million pounds! As you can imagine, not achieving these points will have a large impact on the overall income of a practice. As a result, QOF will often be a driver rather than an outcome. What do I mean? Well, practices cannot afford to lose this income so often they will come at it from the angle of 'What do I need to do to get the points (read: money!)?' rather than 'If I deliver patient care in this area to a high standard then I will also get my QOF points – win-win!' I'll leave other areas of this book to discuss the merits of QOF, but from a financial perspective we know that QOF points are a major part of a practice's income and it is a foolish individual who does not ensure that the maximum amount of points are achieved each year!

The second income stream, enhanced income, is all that lies outside of the core contract. Many practices will actively choose to pursue other income opportunities outside their core contract, and these can be 'enhanced services' – essentially services that either are over and above the core contract or historically may have been provided in secondary care but are now also suited to the primary care environment. Examples are extended hours, anticoagulation clinics, minor surgery, diabetes level 2 and 3 clinics, and pain management/acupuncture. In addition, there may well be private work that GPs choose to take on – simple examples here would be medicals and reports for insurance companies and medical assessments for heavy goods vehicle drivers.

In each case, it is crucial that the practice (usually the business manager) conducts a cost-benefit analysis on any of these optional services. What seems like a great opportunity at first glance can actually be a loss-making activity if costs are not well planned and managed. The tariff will be paid to the practice for each completed service, so time needs to be spent understanding exactly what this means.

It is important to take into account all costs – amazingly, the one area most overlooked is time and skill. Who is going to deliver the service – is it healthcare assistant (HCA), nurse or GP led? How long is each patient appointment? Do we need a new piece of equipment? Is it better to buy it outright or shall we lease it? Does it need calibrating? Again, what costs are involved? How many appointments per annum do we need to break even? What is the maximum output of the service based on capacity and patient list sizes?

As you can see, there are many factors to take into account and each business case needs to be carefully reviewed before a decision is made. It is important to note that the practice may agree to deliver an enhanced service even if the profit from this is minimal *if* the overall benefit is positive. By investing money into a particular area of healthcare the practice may see a related decrease in demand in other areas, with potential savings to be made.

How is money allocated?

Primary income stream (money allocated to the practice)	Secondary income stream (additional to practice-based activity)
Registered list size	Diabetes level 2, including satellite clinics
Practice socio-demographics	Warfarin
Selected cost elements (rates/rents)	Minor operations
QOF	Musculoskeletal clinics
Enhanced services (direct/local)	Electromyogram (EMG) for carpal tunnel syndrome diagnosis
	Pain management
	Training (i.e. GP registrars, medical students)
	Medical examinations and reports

MANAGING COSTS

On the other side of the business to income we have our costs or expenditure. At practice level, the partners are accountable for ensuring that all other costs associated with the day-to-day running of the business are met. Examples of costs are as follows:

- **Salaried colleagues, including National Insurance and pensions** – to keep the practice running there is an army of colleagues including the receptionists, administration team, medical secretaries, healthcare assistants, business/practice manager and not forgetting the salaried GPs. When we talk about salaries, the true cost of an employee is much more. Let's take a salaried GP as an example, earning £70 000 per year. The employer will need to pay employer pension contributions at 14% (£9800), National Insurance at 13.8% after allowances (£7400) and in some cases medical indemnity fees (approximately £6000 for a full-time GP). As you can see, the true cost to the practice is nearer £93 000! The same principles apply to all employees and notionally you can estimate that the true cost of an employee is around 25% more than their base salary.
- **Medical consumables** – another area borne by the practice is consumables. This can be items such as couch rolls, latex gloves, intrauterine devices and so forth. It is very much a worthwhile exercise to shop around for these items and to build up a good relationship with one or two suppliers. It is astounding the difference in costs of these basic items, and your usual supplier may not be as competitive as you think.
- **Utilities (gas/electric)** – a reasonably sized building takes a lot of heating and will have a considerable amount of equipment requiring electricity (such as personal computers, monitors, printers, lighting, automatic doors and even the mundane items such as fridges, kettles, microwaves).

The commercial market for utilities is less competitive than the domestic market, and a medium to large building will cost anywhere in the region of £1000 per month for electricity and between £600 and £800 per month for gas.

- **Telephones** – an essential tool in communicating with our patients and other care providers, but telephones can prove expensive. Most patients now use mobiles, some even at the expense of having a landline. To make matters worse, we have a number of NHS bodies that use the so-called non-geographic numbers beginning with a code of 0844 or similar – these are extremely expensive in comparison with local and national call rates.

- **Insurance** – as owners of the business, the partners will need to ensure they are adequately insured. Some insurance, such as public liability, is a legal requirement; others, such as locum insurance, are optional. However, as with all insurance it is about offsetting the risk against an acceptable cost (i.e. the premium). How much are we prepared to pay to ensure we have a guaranteed income, should a GP or other key employee be off sick for a sustained period of time? Insurance is a competitive area and considerable savings can be made here, particularly if a bespoke/tailored policy is purchased, rather than the off-the-shelf 'one-size-fits-all' products offered by some insurance companies in the healthcare market.

- **Postage** – the number of letters posted each year by a medium-sized practice is in the thousands. Considering the cost of postage stamps, postage can amount to a sizable sum of money, particularly when you include the cost of the envelope, paper and printing! A practice really needs to weigh up the benefits of a franking machine, as the savings currently can be 30% or more per letter sent; however, there needs to be a good volume of postage to deliver savings and offset the cost of leasing or purchasing the franking machine.

- **Out-of-hours care provision** – as part of the core contract, a practice will have a defined set of working hours within which it must provide care for its patients. If a practice decides to close, for example, for regular training each week/month, then it must employ the services of a third-party 'out-of-hours' care provider. All associated costs must be borne by the practice.

- **Accountants** – they tend to charge in many different ways: some charge a fixed amount per partner, some charge by the hour and others charge a percentage of the overall income of a practice. Whichever method is agreed by the partners, the total cost per annum is significant.

These are all examples of areas of cost that the practice is accountable for and that can be a real risk to the business if not managed. There are lots of other examples of costs involved in the running of the business; whether they are regular recurring costs or they are ad hoc, each and every cost needs to be challenged to ensure that it is timely, competitively priced and able to be justified.

Also, as mentioned earlier, anything left in the pot at the end of all of this is profit and it is this that is divided equitably among the partners in the form of a drawing.

> *Money is better than poverty, if only for financial reasons.*
>
> —Woody Allen

General practice business running costs

Partner drawings

Salaried colleagues (including National Insurance and pensions)

Medical consumables

Utilities (gas/electric)

Telephones

Accountants

Insurances

Postage

Out-of-hours care provision

MANAGING THE BUSINESS

Practices employ a manager or, indeed, managers to look after the running of the business, removing the need for the partners to have to deal with the minutiae of the business.

Traditionally a **practice manager** would head this up. These individuals are often time-served individuals, with many having worked for the practice for a good number of years, developing their skills in many progressive roles. These practice managers have strong 'in-house' management and high local knowledge – they are usually The Oracle when it comes to knowing who to contact regarding a particular query or how a specific part of the NHS bureaucracy works!

They are often very good at the operational side of the business. Some of them can handle business development as well, but as general practice has become more complex, finding all the skills needed to manage operations and business development within one person becomes less likely.

A newer type of manager is now becoming more prominent in general practice, the **business development manager**. These individuals tend to have worked for external organisations previously, most likely in the private sector. While often relatively new to the NHS, they bring with them a different skill set: operational excellence, particularly around customer (think patient!) focus, efficiency and cost management. Alongside this these managers often offer a greater level of business acumen and strategic thinking. They are able to better appraise options for change, and cost up proposals and so help partners decide which activities are worthwhile (profits, interest) and which are not (hassle, little income).

Why the change? What we had before was good enough, wasn't it? As discussed earlier in this chapter, the changes within the NHS, both those that we know of and those still over the horizon, will necessitate us managing our practices as true businesses that can stand on their own two feet and compete in what is a challenging environment.

In the future, the current small partnerships we see may have to move into larger groups and think of themselves as 'federations'. We may need to think of ourselves as 'primary medical care service providers' rather than as professional partnerships. In the early 1980s the legal profession underwent a process that led to a series of mergers, consolidations and specialisations. It meant that most lawyers aimed their services to a specialised niche market. General practice in the UK may be about to go in a similar direction. In the future we will need business managers as much as or more than practice managers. Whether we like it or not, practices are going to be talking about their 'business strategies' (you have one already, but you may not have openly called it that) and we will need people to develop these strategies for us. Far-sighted practices are already appointing business managers.

We will see more competition coming from the private sector as large public limited companies move into primary care and aggressively grow their market share.

We will see the clinical commissioning groups develop and evolve. It will be the practices that are financially sound and that have strong leadership and robust strategic direction that will be at the forefront of these changes. These practices will be able to capitalise on the opportunities that are presented, making them even stronger businesses, providing high standards of patient care and an acceptable level of reward to those who contribute, whether as a salaried GP or as a GP partner.

Sadly, those practices that fail to adapt to this emerging world may end up disappearing or being swallowed up in takeovers.

Only the wisest and stupidest of men never change.

—Confucius

Chapter 16

How to handle a complaint

Peter Davies

An action for negligence against a doctor is for him unto a dagger. His professional reputation is as dear to him as his body, perhaps more so, and an action for negligence can wound his reputation as severely as a dagger can his body.

—Lord Denning

Courts, damages, newspapers, and all that sort of thing.

—Sir Lancelot Spratt, *Doctor in the House*

It is Monday morning. You have just arrived in surgery. The practice manager asks if he can have a quiet word with you. 'I'm sorry', he says, 'but do you remember you saw Mrs Wood last week? Her daughter's put a written complaint on my desk this morning.'

THE EMOTIONAL PHASE

How do you feel at this instant? I can guarantee it won't be, 'Great, here's a marvellous opportunity for learning.' You are likely to feel some or all of the following:

- upset
- anger
- sadness
- frustration
- tearful
- fearful

- stressed
- catastrophic
- failure
- want to get the notes and start checking
- want to go home and start again
- want to get even
- want a coffee.

You may well feel a lot of anger and resentment towards the complainant and the patient. The complaint may or may not be fair, but to you at this stage it's damn well unfair, after all you did for them, the ungrateful so-and-so, and so on and so forth. Your emotions will be running high, and while this is entirely natural, it's not entirely an effective place from which to work. Find somewhere to have them safely, have a coffee, and then breathe.

The first thing you need to do is to acknowledge your emotions. Then you need some way of cooling off and parking them safely. You still have the morning surgery to do, however much you may want to go home and hide your tears under your duvet. You need to get yourself back into a frame of mind that allows you to do morning surgery well, and not to pass or transfer your feelings to the other patients, nor to colleagues and staff.

This initial **emotional phase** of your response to the complaint is likely to take 24–48 hours. In this time the practice manager will send an initial acknowledgement, but try not to say anything more. Talking with your colleagues or a call to your medical defence organisation often helps get you calmed down – the sky is not about to fall, you probably have not been negligent, you are not about to get carted off to the GMC, your career is not about to end in total abject failure. Calm down, it's only a complaint.

Complaints are unwelcome and no one enjoys them. Young and new doctors often pick them up for various reasons including inexperience of people (they do not quite know how to handle the particular family as firmly or adroitly as the senior partner does), inexperience of local systems so they make silly mistakes (e.g. sending the patient to the wrong place for their blood test) and, finally, for having the temerity to be different from the lovely old senior partner who had been a perfect GP for the last 30 years. (He hadn't, but the retrospectoscope has a golden halo filter built in.)

Complaints are intrinsically stressful events. You can think of our responses to them as being like those of a patient receiving bad news. Using Elisabeth Kübler-Ross's description of this, we will see stages of complaint handling including anger, grief, jealousy, bargaining and resolution. As already described, your initial response to the complaint is likely to be emotional, particularly involving anger and grief.

I would recommend acknowledging your emotions (just as you would do in return for patients). Once the emotions have calmed down you can then move into the **sorting-out phase** (resolution).

THE SORTING-OUT PHASE

In the sorting-out phase you can look at the complaint and see what the question is that it asks. Complaints vary from the trivial to the clinically serious. They can be usefully considered in the following groups:

● complaints about attitude and manner (communication) – these are usually relatively minor
● allegations of errors in procedure of care
● negligence
● criminal allegations.

Most complaints are about minor upsets and the doctor's manner. They arise after a breakdown in communication. These will usually be resolved by some combination of explanation and apology. Remember that acknowledgement of hurt and an apology is not an admission of liability in the legal sense.

The key point in these minor complaints is to calm the situation down – they are only dangerous if you fail to respond, or if you inflame the situation further. Usually they settle pretty quickly. When you consider the complaint more carefully, it may actually show you an area of your personal practice that needs improving, or it may highlight a flaw in practice systems.

Remember that the doctor who receives the complaint may be far from being the most culpable in the situation.

If a complaint is handled well, and the misunderstanding cleared up you may actually end up building a good future relationship with the complainant. Honesty and providing the right missing information at the right time helps answer the question and build trust and respect.

Most doctors get one or two complaints a year to deal with. In the old days this would not have been so, but times have changed. Complaints are now almost routine, and the only doctor with no complaints has probably retired from practice or died. Knowing how to answer complaints is something we will all need to learn.

WHO SHOULD REPLY TO A COMPLAINT?

The practice manager usually sends an initial acknowledgement regarding the complaint. The formal reply can be made either by the partner in charge of complaints or by the doctor who is complained about. Sometimes it is a good service to a colleague to reply to a complaint on their behalf – the outsider often sees the issues more clearly and is free of personal threat from the complaint.

WHAT SHOULD BE IN THE REPLY?

Either way, the letter of response wants to be respectful (even if respect is not merited) and it should answer the patient's questions (however silly) about their care. It wants to be clear about the circumstances and event in question and it wants to be direct. It wants to be factual, with little or no emotion shown except regret for the patient's suffering (this applies no matter how wounded you personally may be feeling). If the doctor's clinical care was entirely appropriate and correct, then say so. Ideally the letter should leave no open questions and no option or need for people to come back for 'clarification' later on. Ideally it will be 'copper-bottomed', so no solicitor or barrister can later pick holes in it. Check the contents of the letter with colleagues and your medical defence organisation before sending it. Do not rush it or write it too soon after the original letter of complaint has come in. Read it again 24 hours later before finally signing it and posting it.

SITUATIONS TO BE WARY OF

Families in grief after a relative has died are particularly likely to initiate complaints as part of their grief and while trying to make sense of what has happened to their loved one. On the medical wards I picked up a dictum that 'it's not a good idea to serve up an unexpected corpse to the family'. Sam Weller in *The Pickwick Papers* reminds us to 'Be wery careful o'vidders'.

Specific clinical allegations are potentially serious; they need careful consideration and a good rebuttal and explanation if you can provide one, or a swift acknowledgement and apology if you are in the wrong. Speak to your colleagues (many practices have a lead complaint partner who reviews complaints and checks replies) or to your medical defence organisation before answering such allegations.

Remember that what is remarkable about general practice is not how often we get it wrong but, rather, how often we get it wrong and are not called to account for it. (And also how often we get it right, sometimes despite ourselves and our interventions.) Doctors with good communication skills may get away with quite serious errors, as long as they keep the family onside and well informed about the events in question. Doctors with poor communication skills need to get things right, as they are likely to attract complaints if they get it wrong.

Complaints are currently more dangerous that negligence allegations. More serious still are allegations of misconduct that may reach the GMC. GMC allegations are dangerous. However, most of the complaints to the GMC fail to meet their threshold for further investigation. The GMC is looking for either exceptionally awful behaviour (usually criminal) or a pattern of poor performance sustained across many cases and settings. It is very unlikely that you would be removed for one bad clinical case. If the GMC did this, then there would not be a single doctor left practising. Most proven examples of poor performance such as negligence actions do not even reach the GMC. The GMC is only interested in what used to be known as 'serious professional misconduct' and what is now described as a significant breach of the principles of good medical practice. You may know if you have done that. The GMC does receive quite a lot of minor complaints, but it tries to turn these back to local complaint channels. The GMC has no interest in investigating these complaints, unless they are an opening to a wider or deeper problem with a professional's performance.

The GMC is sometimes misused in employment disputes between employers and doctors, and it is not a good venue to determine such disputes.

The GMC is not particularly interested in a doctor's views, beliefs or opinions, unless these interfere with their ability to care for patients. The basic rule is that you are entitled to your opinion but not to afflict a patient with it, or to use it to prevent a patient from accessing care. You may have a conscientious or moral objection to a legally sanctioned and available treatment (abortion is the common example here). That is fine, provided you pass the patient to someone else who will provide the care.

The GMC is interested in the doctor who is a severe risk to the safety of patients. The GMC assessment of a case is detailed, and ruled by procedure. Its assessment may well involve occupational health and professional capacity tests, as well as the evidence about the index event in the case. The GMC has ways of dealing with health issues that often manage to protect the patients from harm, and allow the doctor to be rehabilitated. The GMC is, as far as possible in a legal setting, not a vindictive organisation: it wants to sort out serious performance issues if possible and ensure patient safety, not to erase doctors from its register.

Although we are all scared of a GMC case against us, we need to remember that the glue holding doctors to the GMC register is usually far stronger than the forces trying to remove us from it.

LEARNING FROM COMPLAINTS

Most complaints pass by harmlessly enough. They may be wearing at the time. But in time they can come to be seen as useful, and even as an opportunity to learn something. Sadly, they are now a pretty routine part of medical practice and I doubt you will avoid them for long.

In my own career (22 years so far) I have had to answer various minor complaints, two allegations of negligence (both failed) and one GMC complaint (dropped after preliminary enquiries were completed). I cannot say I have enjoyed these, but I have learned from them and I can now use this experience to good effect. As so often in biology and medicine, what does not kill us makes us stronger.

COMPLAINTS AND YOUR APPRAISAL

Declaring the complaints you have received are part and parcel of appraisals. All doctors get complaints and they are there to learn from; you need to show to your appraiser that you have considered each complaint and that you have moved forward to become (it is to be hoped) a more learned doctor as a result. Books have been written with titles such as *Why I'm Right . . . and Everyone Else is Wrong* (by Tom Harris) and *Don't Fix Me, I'm Not Broken* (by Sally Patton); chances are, if you adopt their stances you're in for a roller coaster of unwelcome dramas.

With each complaint you get, ask yourself the following questions:

- Was there anything in my actions that was a catalyst for this?
- Do I need to change any of my actions, attitudes or knowledge to avoid this happening again?
- Was there anything I could have done differently to prevent this?

Our personalities don't always fall in line with those of our patients. As the saying goes, 'You can't please all the people all the time'. Still, working to excel in our communication skills, we can learn to diffuse conflict and, it is to be hoped, to avoid the dramas, even if we don't get on with some of our patients.

FALLING OUT WITH PATIENTS

The basic rule in medicine is to, as far as possible, stay on friendly terms with everyone you meet and avoid falling out with them. The other way of thinking of this is the proposition that a gentleman is never rude to anyone . . . unless he means to be.

So, a useful rule is to never fall out with a patient or partner unless you deliberately mean to do so. In our practice we have sometimes collectively decided to remove some particularly awkward patients from our list. We do not do this often (we have 10 900 patients and this happens less than twice a year), but it is sometimes necessary to ensure smooth running of the practice, and to prevent one patient from monopolising its services unfairly. We did have to answer a complaint from one patient we chose to remove from our list, although we knew to expect this and were ready for it.

CREDIT FROM PATIENTS

Although in this chapter we are talking about the sadness of complaints, remember that we also get many plaudits from our patients. As a general rule, 80% of your use to the patient is your clinical knowledge. However, about 80% of the praise you will ever get will come because of your good communication with and ability to transmit compassion to your patient.

Dr Chris Manning has suggested that we should move to audit and plaudit as simultaneous activities, and I wish we could implement his idea in the NHS. If we are to live in a feedback world then we should get the good alongside the bad, and provide easily accessible routes for both.

Humans are primed to notice what is wrong or different in situations and not to notice how much is well organised and right, which therefore allows the problem to stand out as abnormal. For doctors we need to keep reminding ourselves about how much we get right, and never allow one awkward or poor case to stand for the whole of our practice. As the Reverend Eli Jenkins puts it in *Under Milk Wood*, 'We are not wholly bad or good' and we have to hope that our good outweighs our bad. For most doctors the balance of good over bad is massively in favour of the good.

PERPETRATORS, VICTIMS AND RESCUERS: THE TRIANGULAR DANCE IN COMPLAINTS

One useful way of looking at complaints is to use the framework provided by Dr Stephen Karpman in transactional analysis. He described what is known as the perpetrator victim rescuer triangle (also known as the drama triangle). In the model, everyone in the drama is playing one of three roles: perpetrator, victim or rescuer. Only one of the players can occupy any one role at any time. The drama comes as the players switch between the roles. It is a surprisingly accurate map for many varied situations. It works well even when the drama being studied has more than three players. Even in situations where there are fewer than three players the people involved still tend to generate the three roles. It is as though the roles somehow have to exist. Allow me to elaborate.

If we think of a football match, then team A attack team B. They try to get the ball into team B's net. They foul team B. The referee steps in to rescue team B from the unfair attack. Team A now feel they are the victim of the referee's attack on them. The referee thought he was being a caretaker. Team B move to support the referee and his actions, thereby becoming the rescuers. At each stage the participants are moving swiftly among the various roles in the triangle.

In medicine, doctors are usually the rescuers, the patient is the victim, and the attack has been perpetrated by disease in some form or other. The doctor is there to rescue the patient from their attacker. The doctor has a duty to be the rescuer. They may feel a failure when they cannot effect the rescue. The patient may well be disappointed that the rescue had not gone to plan, so then the patient complains about the doctor, and now the doctor feels like the victim of the patient's attack. Phrases such as 'after all I had done for them' and such like come out. Various people act as rescuers: the colleagues and staff who comfort the doctor who has been complained about, the relatives comforting the one who has initiated the complaint, the medical defence trying to diffuse the situation. A lot of people are acting very quickly and moving around the different roles of perpetrator, victim and caretaker very rapidly. The situation is unstable and has potential for drama.

In nature a triangular shape is a very strong one. In human relationships triangles are intrinsically unbalanced, as can be seen in these examples of common triangular situations:

- good cop, bad cop and suspect
- defence, prosecution and judge
- wife, husband and mistress
- team A, team B and referee
- persecutor, victim and rescuer
- doctor, patient and illness
- thesis, antithesis, synthesis.

In these scenarios more generally:

- The **perpetrator** can be seen as the agonist for change, the attacker, the initiator, the innovator, the doer, the one who *disturbs the equilibrium.*
- The **victim** can be seen as the recipient of change, the passive one, the damaged one, the one *whose equilibrium is disturbed*, the reactor, and the antagonist to change.
- The **rescuer** is acting as someone who tries to damp down the excesses of the perpetrator and *restore the equilibrium* of the triangle. The rescuer acts to take care of both victim and perpetrator.

Unfortunately, the stabilising forces that the rescuer can bring to bear on the other two forces interact variably with the other forces in motion and so may or may not achieve balance. Indeed, a stabilising force applied at the wrong moment can perpetuate another round of imbalance, this time with the would-be rescuer becoming the perpetrator! Karpman described beautifully the dramatic switches the players in the drama triangle made as they swapped between their apparently allotted roles.

As you experience a complaint, think of this model and reflect on where you are at one time within it. You may be feeling that you are a victim, but are you actually attacking? You may be thinking you are rescuing, but are you actually subtly attacking your colleague's abilities? (For example, are you sure you got your communication right that day? Mrs Wood is usually easy-going.)

Dr David Ryland, a respected and now retired GP educator for Calderdale, UK, commented when I used it as a metaphor in a *BMJ* letter, 'It's a great description, but how do you get out of the triangle?' I am not sure that we ever do leave this triangle. My suspicion is that we stop it oscillating too wildly, and after a while we move on to another triangle somewhere else.

Variable	Caretaker/ rescuer	Persecutor/ perpetrator	Victim
Some positions and attitudes a doctor can occupy in the drama triangle	Caring for patients Learned Rescues patients from disease Cares at whatever cost to him/herself or his/her own life	Negligence Attacking politicians over lack of funds Judging patients 'worthy' or 'unworthy' Anger at a patient's or management's idiocy Afflicting patients with health (e.g. excessive health promotion)	Of a complaint: 'After all I did for him, how could he?' Of politicians: 'If they knew what was going on here, down at ground level' Of managers: 'What do bean counters know about running a hospital? If they were any good they'd not be working in the NHS' Of other doctors: 'Why am I always the only one left behind to pick up the pieces of other people's work?' Of patient demand: 'There's just too many people with nothing better to do than worry about their bodies' Of the press: 'Courts, papers . . . hmm . . . very bad'
Some positions and attitudes a patient can occupy	And how are you today, doctor? 'I'm sorry to bother you with this' 'When there's others worse off than me'	Attack on doctor via complaint system 'If you don't do something doctor, there'll be a price to pay' 'I'm not seeing that Paki doctor' Of themselves, afflicting themselves with ill health	Patient a victim . . . of disease of negligent acts of poor service of underfunding and waiting lists of their own mistakes (incidents, trauma, tobacco and alcohol) of their 'metabolism' or 'genes'
Some positions regulators can take	'There's a problem here and we will fix it' Not their patients, but my voters Crusader for quality and public services	Blame someone else Denigrate professional standards as special pleading Say anything for a good headline Comment freely on other people's affairs	'Typical, they're always after money' 'Patients are more loyal to their doctor than to their MP' 'The press will say anything' 'There's no point in giving them extra beds, they'll only find patients to block them with' 'Events, dear boy, events'

CLINICAL NEGLIGENCE

The defence organisations now treat negligence as separate events from complaints. Surprisingly, they rarely overlap. Negligence actions are a specific event initiated by the patient's solicitor and decided on the basis of the facts of the case and the expert opinion about those facts. They tend to be specific allegations, and they usually allege one of the following:

- failure to see the patient
- failure to properly assess the patient
- failure to make the right diagnosis
- failure to make the right treatment choice
- failure to make a referral onward
- failure to warn about untoward consequences such as side effects of treatment.

Remember that to establish a negligence claim from a complaint, the claimant (through their solicitor) has to show:

- a duty of care exists
- breach of that duty
- quantifiable harm has arisen from the breach.

It is surprising how rarely the lawyers manage to prove this. Remember that the standard of practice expected is that of a reasonable other doctor, not that of a 'top expert'. You may have made a mistake, but as long as it is easily made and others in a similar position could make the same mistake, then it is within the normal limits of professional practice.

Negligence actions very rarely end in court, or generating publicity. Most are either rejected, where the claim has no merit, or settled, where the claim has some merit. There is a group in the middle where the case is arguable either way. Even these rarely end up in court, with most being settled by a meeting of experts (medical and legal) before a trial.

Very few cases go to court, and this is good for doctors as it avoids the stress of a court appearance, and it avoids the risks of a doctor's evidence being picked apart by a barrister. Courts are risky places, and a court case going wrong is a severe risk to one's reputation. The Lord's Prayer includes 'Do not bring us to the time of trial' – most negligence lawyers and medical defence organisations say 'Amen' to that. A negligence action may offend your professional conscience, and you may want to fight it all the way. The medical defence organisations tend to take a wider view about what is fully defensible and whether the fight is valuable, either to their individual member or to our profession as a whole. The costs and risks of a day in court are so high that often discretion is the better part of valour.

Negligence actions rarely lead to professional conduct proceedings. They are seen as actions about mistakes and hazards of practice, rather than as events that raise questions about the doctor's professional standing. The settlement agreed is between doctor and patient, and usually the issue stops at that point. There is no duty on the doctor to tell anyone else about the outcome of the case. In particular, there is no current duty for the doctor to mention the case or its settlement to their medical director or clinical commissioning group. Negligence actions and their outcomes may well provide good learning for your appraisal discussion, but even here some doctors will just file them under experience.

Finally, remember that although the unfortunate doctor who is the subject of the allegations does not usually do well out of the case, there are likely to be other doctors acting as expert witnesses who actually may earn and learn well from the case. It's an ill wind that blows nobody some good.

SUMMARY

Complaints are stressful for doctors and they are not particularly enjoyable. They have two main components: your emotional reaction and the facts of the case that allow it to be sorted out. You need to pay attention to both parts. Once you get through the emotional phase of dealing with a complaint and come to the sorting-out phase, then some learning is possible. However, it is a rough school of teaching and a somewhat bitter experience. Help and advice from colleagues in the practice and at medical defence organisations is very useful and should be taken freely. Remember, although it may be your turn this week, time moves on and next week it may be you helping out a colleague.

Summary points for dealing with a complaint

Talk to your colleagues

If the nature is more serious, talk to your defence organisation

Give time for the emotional response to settle

Reflect on what went wrong

Work with the practice manager and/or the senior partner to diffuse the situation with a response

Use this unpleasant situation as a learning experience to examine your clinical practice and communication skills for future scenarios

---

REFERENCES

1 Wikipedia. *Karpman Drama Triangle.* Available at: http://en.wikipedia.org/wiki/Karpman_drama_triangle (accessed 17 December 2011).
2 Karpman SB. *Fairy Tales and Script Drama Analysis.* Available at: www.karpman dramatriangle.com/pdf/DramaTriangle.pdf (accessed 3 April 2012).
3 www.KarpmanDramaTriangle.com (accessed 17 December 2011).

Chapter 17

How to deal with your heart sinking

Peter Davies

Heartsink patients are a special category. The phenomenon is a real one, but the label is not an objective one. **The heart that sinks is the *doctor's*, in response to the thought or presence of a particular patient.** It is a mixed cognitive and affective feeling for the doctor, and it is usually not pleasant. We all have some heartsink patients, and they drain our resources, often for little return on the time and effort they suck out from us. Heartsink patients are so, not because of the clinical difficulty they present (most of us manage complexity and co-morbidity quite well, and enjoy a clinical challenge) but usually because of the feeling they induce that they are consuming our resources, freely and greedily, and we despair of ever stopping what is an unfair trade. After seeing a heartsink patient the doctor will feel stressed, exhausted and fragile, and this will be an emotional drain rather than a clinical challenge to the doctor. Heartsink patients are usually unaware that they have this effect, and they persist despite many signals that others would have picked up on. Indeed, a heartsink patient's ability to ignore the minimal cues from the doctor is almost a defining feature of his or her lack of insight.

There are **four common groups** of heartsink patients.

1. The dependent clinger: while thanking the doctor for all they've done, the patient is desperate for reassurance and shows this by returning repeatedly with an array of symptoms.
2. The entitled demander: this patient views the doctor as a barrier to receiving services and complains if every request is not met.
3. The manipulative help-rejector: has a quenchless need for emotional supplies and returns repeatedly to tell the doctor the treatment did not work.
4. The self-destructive denier – although possibly suffering from serious disease makes no alteration in lifestyle. It seems to the doctor that the patient's aim is to defeat any attempts to preserve his life.

All of these patients will take up a lot of time and only induce frustration in their doctors. Somehow their behaviour will make the doctor move away from wanting to help the patient and towards a place where all they want to do is to get the patient out of their room. The effort the patient puts into wanting 'help' and 'services' is matched only by their inability to ever follow through on any plan or to attend appointments arranged. They hang around the consulting room wanting something, but not anything we could actually provide. They often want an instantaneous external solution to something that is actually an internal character flaw. They show a level of personal ineffectiveness that is not justified by any pathology or its consequences. They resist any attempt at gaining understanding of their problems or at using the understanding they have. They will complain about being disempowered, while all the while handing over ever more control of their lives to experts they do not really need.

I think the heartsink phenomenon **goes beyond medicine**. I think that in life generally there are some people who make our hearts sink and some who make our hearts sing for joy. I suspect that retailers have heartsink customers, and that teachers have many heartsink children and parents. I suspect the description can be reversed, and that some patients will have heartsink doctors – a doctor they do not like, whose judgement they don't trust, or who offended them or their family in the past. The patient's heart would sink if offered an appointment with that doctor. At the medical regulatory level, a heartsink doctor for a medical director is one who shows no insight into the possibility that his or her performance may be impaired and who persists on repeating the same mistake while still insisting he or she is right.

There are various ways of dealing with such patients. First, you need to recognise your own feelings. These may be intense and unpleasant, but you cannot show that to the patient. You may have got the scenario wrong, or you may need more information or to get a better diagnosis, so try to get enough information to define the problem accurately. Sometimes in this attempt the understanding needed emerges. Sometimes the opposite happens, and the more you converse the less the problem is defined and the more a diffuse mess emerges.

Then if you can, and however much you may not feel like doing so, try to build some rapport with the patient. Find some redeeming feature about the patient, even if this is simply a pet dog or cat. Listen attentively, use empathy, avoid confrontation and make eye contact (except with aggressors). Create a shared understanding of the problem, if you can, although this is easier to say than achieve. Even when you think you have achieved a shared understanding, heartsink patients may either swap doctor or change the plan unilaterally.

Encourage the patient to take responsibility for his or her *own* health – although one of the classic characteristics of heartsink patients is that they try to turn their problems into your problems, rather than doing anything about it themselves.

Create a shared management plan. Use patient diaries and other methods to help patients gain an insight into linking illness with psychosocial events. Provide a firm, structured, consistent approach, and alert your colleagues across the practice to what you are doing.

Communicate with other doctors – sing from the same hymn sheet. Avoid doctor shopping (i.e. where the patient sees many doctors to get a variety of opinions, investigations, referrals and treatments). Young doctors should be particularly wary about being approached by patients wanting 'a new view on the problem'.

Discuss with your colleagues – some patients make everyone's heart sink. Sometimes your colleagues may have useful extra background information that will make the situation more understandable, or they may have experience in having handled a similar situation in the past. Sometimes a kind colleague will take your heartsink patient off you, although this may be a trade rather than pure altruism. The generous response to such an action is to say thank you and then accept one of his or her heartsink patients in return.

Always keep control of the situation. Whose problem is it? Partially yours, and maybe the patient's as well. Housekeep yourself, so that the negative emotions do not transfer to you or your family . . . transferring these emotions to others is unfair.

Finally, remember to celebrate **the heart sing patients** – the ones you like, the ones you enjoy seeing and the ones who give you a lift when you see them, so that you enjoy the person while you are treating their disease. Most GPs do actually like people. There are actually many more patients we like and enjoy helping than there are heartsink patients.

If you ask me to put numbers on all this I would say that, on average, out of 100 patients seen by me, 90 patients are straightforward and ask sensible questions along the lines of 'Doctor, please may I have some help with my problem?' About five patients are medically complex – that is, you need to think hard about the complex medicine involved in these cases and strike some fine balances between over- and undertreatment, benefits versus risks and so on. These cases are difficult, but they are what we really earn our money on. Finally, about five cases involve patients who are just awkward – something about them means that they need firm handling, or there is a knack to knowing how to handle these patients. These patients benefit most from continuity and consistency. If you want to see why, see how much your colleagues struggle with them when you go on holiday.

Even with heartsink patients there is an argument for keeping the ones you know and with whom you have reached some kind of equilibrium. Unless they go too far and become offensive or aggressive, then, once you have worked them out, most of the hard work is done. If you take them off your list you may find your colleague down the road has them allocated to him, and responds by sending some of his own up to you. And they may be even worse.

Chapter **18**

Mentorship

Lindsay Moran

We all have mentors (whether or not we appreciate them as that) who we can turn to in our professional and personal lives. They are the people we look up to, whose advice we value and who we turn to when we need help. Our mentors will change over time: the person who is an appropriate mentor to us as a house officer may not necessarily be the same person to go to for advice when it comes to accepting your first GP partnership role, for instance. The type of mentor can vary too: we can have mentors who operate on a small, personal scale – those we talk to frequently, such as our peers, our family and the considerate soul who listens to us talk at the end of a working day about our heartsinks. Then there are those older and wiser mentors whose experience and knowledge we yearn to have a piece of, who we perhaps speak to less often but who we turn to with large, important matters such as which career path to take or how to overcome difficult obstacles.

Mentors are all very individual to our needs. It is usually the mentee to choose the mentor, rather than the other way around. It is to be hoped that when you are allocated a formal mentor, such as your vocational training schemes (VTS) trainer for instance, they will be someone who will be a good mentor to you and with whom you get along, although this is not always the case, unfortunately.

Outside of formal allocations, mentors will usually come our way by chance interactions, workplace encounters or perhaps as friends of friends. You might even be more proactive and seek out a mentor based on the reputation of that person. However you find a mentor, the key to getting the most out of the mentorship process is how useful they are and how we utilise them.

Experience is something that takes time. Nobody gains the title of 'Expert: been there, done that, got the T-shirt' without pulling out a few hairs or banging their head on a few tables. Gaining experience is a frustrating process. To become a GP we will have had to do jobs we didn't like, worked hours that made us grumpy, sat in on weekends to revise for exams, been walked over by bosses or nurses and made a lot of mistakes that cost us a lot of time and probably money too. Wouldn't it be great if someone had taken us by the hand and walked us through that process? Well, that can never happen; we need to have made our own mistakes and learned from them to become who we are today. However, a mentor can guide you around a few of the potholes, point out the oasis in the distance and, it is to be hoped, make the trip a much more savoury experience.

ROYAL COLLEGE OF GENERAL PRACTITIONERS AND MENTORSHIP

Sometimes you haven't met a mentor who can fulfil your career needs, other times it may be because you move to a new area and you don't know anyone locally. In these situations, being introduced to a mentor can be very helpful.

With the First5® initiative, the RCGP has launched a mentor scheme on their website. It works like a nice online dating system: you provide your details as a mentee (someone looking for a mentor), read through the list of available mentors and their attributes, find someone who seems to most suit your personality and career needs and then select to hook up. Even if you already have a mentor, extra diversity and perspective can be gained by having two or more mentors.

Lindsay's experience

What Peter wrote about in Chapter 13, about isolation after the VTS certainly rings true. I first worked as a locum after qualification. You sometimes feel like an anonymous person, walking into a strange surgery at your specified time to simply do your job and then leave. Unless you work somewhere regularly and then slowly build up your relationships, it can be very isolating. After a period of locuming I took on a couple of maternity locums and this made life easier. You get to mix and form a rapport with the team, and this also makes it easier to approach people there when you have uncertainties.

What I found after the VTS is that without your designated clinical and educational trainers, you start to look to other people for mentorship – indeed, the RCGP First5® supports this as one of its pillars. Depending on where you are in your life, what you are looking for and whom you come across, you need a variety of mentors to suit your various needs.

I have been indebted to numerous people who have fulfilled this role for me in a personal and professional setting. Prior to my specialty training, there was my trainer Dr Jane Petty, an incredibly enthusiastic and cheerful GP in Bradford. At a time of career crossroads she described to me what a delightful career general practice can be and told me to go for it. I am also indebted to my VTS trainers: Dr Simon Hall, a portfolio GP, with his daily humour, gave me optimism and helped me through my initial career doubts; and Dr Sarah Hutchinson, a GP so popular with the patients, a calm clinician to observe, who handled all situations with seeming ease. She cemented for me that I had made the correct career choice. Both despaired at my begrudging approach to the ePortfolio, but their persistence got me through it in the end. Now, in the absence of a trainer, I tend to find that with each new job one or two doctors stand out as being a clinical mentor, although I try not to overburden any one person with this. Without the trainer security blanket I have made so many more phone calls to the hospitals to chat my cases through with the registrars and consultants.

Over time my co-author Dr Peter Davies has unofficially become my mentor. I met him initially at the RCGP Yorkshire Faculty, when he was the chair, controlling a room around a menacingly large boardroom table, and I was a registrar who felt intimidated to even open my mouth (although that soon changed!). Peter has produced the bulk of this book in whirlwind time with extreme dedication . . . despite being a full-time GP partner, member of the RCGP Council, an appraisal lead, the Yorkshire provost, a prolific author and a husband and father – the list is exhausting to even write! He describes me as a scattergun with my ideas and plans, with a lack of focus. That's true, and fine for now. I struggle to say 'no' when an opportunity presents itself, but hopefully over time my efforts will be fine-tuned from random firing to more accurate, focused, constructive achievements. Peter has been helpful to me by providing the voice of experience for a variety of needs including up-and-coming jobs, publications and writing this book. It really has been invaluable to have someone skilled and approachable to go to for life advice.

My partner, Dr Mahesh Jayaram, is a Psychiatrist and another person with a list as long as your arm of additional hats and roles. Every day I get home and ask, 'How was your day, honey?' and then feel jealous and amazed that he seems to get through 10 times the number of tasks in a day that I could even write a list on. Like other people who carry the title 'experienced', when he has a job to do, he puts his head down and gets on and does it. He delegates to his administration staff and juniors and he prioritises. This all sounds obvious and sensible, but it takes experience to be able to actually put these points into action. He has also been an invaluable source of life consultation and stress-relieving debriefs.

When thinking to future mentors, I had my first appraisal this year and, although I don't know him very well, I chose Dr Richard Vautrey as my appraiser. I attend the Leeds Local Medical Committee, which Dr Vautrey is a member of, and I have also been to other talks that he has given on the White Paper. Needless to say, every time I open the newspaper I read the comments that he made to reporters, defending the hard work of GPs. I admire how he seems to juggle 100 roles simultaneously, as I struggle with distractions and procrastination, and I admire the fact that he speaks with such a polished air of authority. Consequently, I thought he would be a great person to overview my achievements and give me advice.

My parents are not medics, and the advice I get from them is often in direct contrast with the advice I get elsewhere, but who else is better to guide you than someone who has known you your whole life? Their advice is that I work too hard. I always seem to be busy and on the go and they think I should give myself more rest. They have my best interests at heart. This is thoughtful advice, and I do like my holidays and time off; however, I also think that while you have the time, energy and opportunities you should make hay while the sun shines!

On the flipside, I now work as a tutor for third- and fourth-year university students. It's a great role. Aside from making you feel a little mature, it makes you realise what valuable skills and experience you possess to guide others along their career and life paths. I know many of them won't need me once they qualify, but there is something lovely about being able to help others develop.

Chapter 19

Learning points

Peter Davies

In this chapter I have gathered together some thoughts, reflections and ideas that I have picked up over time and which I have found useful. I am grateful to the many people who have drawn my attention to these points. The points are presented here only briefly but be aware that they are punchy. They are quite provocative, and they may well spark some reflection and debate – this is good. I hope you will find them useful at various times in your career, or even just for your amusement and consideration. Although some of these have been mentioned at other points in this book, I think it is useful to present them here as a stand-alone list.

PREVALENCE AND INCIDENCE

- **Demand is like cholesterol.** Blood cholesterol reflects two things: how much is in our diet and how our liver handles it. Likewise, demand for medical appointments depends on the incidence of symptoms and on what doctors do with those symptoms.
- In a GP setting the incidence of symptoms is far greater than that of pathology. Biomedicine occurs at the intersection of the iceberg of disease with the iceberg of symptoms. Many, maybe most, symptoms have no pathological significance. Many diseases have no specific symptoms. Being able to negotiate this intersection without saying 'phaeochromocytoma' too often is a great ability.
- It is more important to be right about ruling out pathology than it is to be right about exactly what pathology is present. (You can get the hospital doctors to do that for us.)
- Time will tell for most things, but if it is likely to tell you all too quickly, admit the patient acutely.

- The good doctor may refer more or less, as he or she knows a lot of medicine. The bad doctor may also refer more or less, as he or she knows too little medicine. Therefore, referral rates are no guide to the quality of the referring doctor.
- If a popular doctor leaves a surgery, consultation rates often drop. If a popular doctor joins a surgery, consultation rates go up. Demand for appointments is in part a popularity marker of the doctor. Demand for appointments is only partly explained by the incidence of pathology.

By pulling all these points together we reach a conclusion that **prevalence depends on what you do with incidence!**

WHY GPs WORK

GPs are apparently poor at much biomedicine. It seems that each week there is yet another demonstration of GP inadequacy for one severe disease or another. We miss diagnoses; we underprescribe some drugs and overprescribe others; we commit errors of omission and commission. We may be ideally placed to spot many things and yet we seem to be singularly good at not spotting them. *Nunc dimittis*: we ask for remission of our many sins. Despite this, however, the late Barbara Starfield's research work in the United States and elsewhere shows that employing GPs reduces the mortality rate in an area.[1] We actually work! The more focused on primary care a healthcare system is, the lower the overall mortality rate is in an area.

How can these facts be squared up?

Sometimes GPs are not great at biomedicine; even when we are, the successes of biomedicine are often technical interventions such as major operations, cancer treatments, magnetic resonance imaging scanners and so forth, and these are all done in specialised settings, usually within hospitals. That is, as GPs we are often the conduits to the best of biomedicine.

I think GPs work for an entirely different reason. Aaron Antonovsky, a medical sociologist from New York and Be'er Sheva, turns talk about health on its head, away from disease avoidance and treatment.[2] He describes 'salutogenesis' – that is, the positive generation of health. He says that healthy people have a 'sense of coherence' that enables them to handle the slings and arrows of outrageous fortune well, without undue stress or disease development.

A good network of family, friends and other helpful contacts boosts the sense of coherence. At the social level this concept is commonly called 'social capital'. The knowledge that there is a local doctor and a reliable medical service that can help you when needed adds to the social capital of an area. So too does good transport, jobs, clean surroundings and low crime rates. The presence of GPs may work, as it helps people develop their sense of coherence via social capital.

The presence of and relationship with (but not necessarily the use of) GPs may be salutogenic.

One consequence of this theory is that when social capital falls, the incidence of both symptoms and pathology will rise, and therefore the use of GP services will also rise. The Polish immigrants with their 'untier syndrome' after the Second World War exemplify this relationship well. When they got settled, their sense of coherence improved and their social capital rose and so it stopped hurting quite so much here . . . unt here.

One-sentence summary of this section: **It is unlikely that the effectiveness of general practice and primary care is entirely down to its biomedical agency.**

THE ROSE PARADOX

The Rose paradox is named after the English epidemiologist Geoffrey Rose.[3] It explains that a small change made over a large population at risk will make little difference to any one person in that population but will make a huge difference to the overall illness experience of that population. For example, if you were treating a specific patient with hypertension, a 5 mmHg drop in systolic blood pressure would not be sufficient to reduce his or her risk of cardiovascular events significantly, but reducing average systolic blood pressure in our country by 5 mmHg would give a large reduction in the incidence of stroke and myocardial infarction. Conversely, a big change in the health status of an individual person in a population has little effect on the overall health or illness of the host populations. For example, performing a heart transplant on a patient with cardiomyopathy is of great benefit to that patient but it has little impact on the overall population health.

The Rose paradox shows that the population perspective and the individual patient perspective are different. The problem is that most of our medical evidence comes from studies of populations rather than narratives of individual cases. However, most day-to-day medical practice is concerned with the unfolding of medical events in individual patients' cases. Also, as humans we have a better ear for narrative and people than we do for abstract notions of risk and large numbers of individuals in a population. Knowing whether you are using a population-based approach or an individual-based approach is crucial to applying medical evidence accurately. Both viewpoints have merit, but it takes discernment to understand and synthesise the insight of both. The divergence between perspectives of population and individual doctors and patients cannot be bridged by 'better implementation of evidence'. Fundamental differences between these perspectives are not easy to reconcile, either intellectually or practically.

This leads me to be wary when people call for better integration of general practice and public health – the approach to an individual is different from that to a population. What is good for one may not be good for many. What is good for many may not be good for some individuals. This question of the good, and whose good we should be looking out for, leads to the two great ethical systems of deontology and utilitarianism that exist in tension throughout the NHS and in every consultation. Too few people understand this paradox, yet it is a fault line that runs through all medical evidence and those who do not understand it make major errors of perspective and interpretation.

One-sentence summary of this section: **A small change across many individuals at risk will achieve more improvement in health (disease avoidance) than will treating one person with a major illness.**

In wider terms, it is the medical version of the philosophical problem of how to balance fairly between the one and the many.

THE ROSE QUESTION

This question is attributed to Dr Eric Rose, a recently retired GP and well-respected senior member of the British Medical Association's General Practitioners Committee. This question is one every senior partner and local medical committee officer needs to know. When as a GP you find yourself being asked to do something and you are not sure about it, or you are not sure whether it is actually your job to do it or not, then this question often sorts the dilemma out. The question is: 'Would you like to show me where in my terms of service, or any other agreement, it says that I am required to do that?'

Usually whoever is asking you to do something you don't think you need to do or should do will scarper rapidly at this point. However, if they can show you the relevant paragraph then you will need to back down gracefully.

Knowing your terms of service is a dry but important task. Doctors who get into trouble often do so because they do not know the specific requirements of their contract.

THE 80/20 RULE (THE PARETO PRINCIPLE)[4]

Life is not fair, and some people achieve more in an hour of work than others do. Much more. The 80/20 rule describes this phenomenon – the principle of asymmetric reward and effort. It was first noted by Pareto, an economist in northern Italy, in relation to land and money distribution, and has been found in many other scenarios and settings since his original description.

The 80/20 rule crops up in many guises in general practice.

- 20% of your patients will take 80% of your appointments.
- 80% of your stress will come from 20% of your patients.
- Within that 20% of patients, 80% of problems will come from 20% of them.

If you need to reduce your stress levels, look at that small group of patients (4%).

As a GP I summarise this as in any group of 100 patients I treat:
- 90% are straightforward.
- 5% are medically awkward – the medicine itself is complex.
- About 5% are flipping awkward!

Other examples include:
- 80% of exam marks are gathered quickly. Have you covered the basics well? Do you need to bother about the remaining 20%?
- 80% of your Quality and Outcomes Framework score is gathered easily. How much time and effort should you spend on the final 20%?
- 20% of causes give 80% of outcomes.
- 20% of inputs create 80% of outputs.

The 80/20 rule is actually a superb statement of the asymmetry of reward and effort. If you know how to use it to your advantage, it increases your effectiveness and allows you to rapidly steer clear of high-hassle, low-reward work and projects. It also supports the idea that you should acknowledge and delegate your weaker areas of activity – someone else will be glad of the work, and he or she will do this work more enthusiastically and more efficiently than you. In return, you can then do more of what you are more effective at doing.

This is a superb rule to know for time management purposes. It allows you to prioritise well and to quickly sort material into the four groups, or spheres of action, outlined in Stephen Covey's time management model:[5]
1. Urgent and unimportant
2. Urgent and important
3. Not urgent, important
4. Not urgent, not important.

When you can do this well you work out what you can put on your 'to-stop-doing list' and concentrate on those bits where you are effective and efficient. Let the other bits go, either to someone else or to nowhere at all.

The 80/20 rule summarises just how unfair life can be. If you learn to use it well you become one of the 20% of people who run off with 80% of the reward – all for simply understanding a little gearing – leaving the plodders wondering in your wake.

GOODHART'S LAW

When a measure becomes a target it ceases to be a measure.

Charles Goodhart, a central banker, first described Goodhart's law.[6] In these target-driven days of medicine, Goodhart's law is a useful rule to know. You can use it to surprise primary care trust managers very well. It is a statement of Albert Einstein's quote, 'Everything that can be counted does not necessarily count; everything that counts cannot necessarily be counted.'

We live in a world of avid measurers. Researchers, managers, ministers and many others want numerical data on all sorts of things. You will fill your appraisal folder with lots of these sets of data. Do any of them actually mean anything? Are they accurately measured? Do they measure what matters?

Think before you measure anything, and remember the joiner's maxim 'measure twice, cut once'.

If you want more fun with this idea, try my piece (with Dr Adrian Kenny) on 'probophilia' – the pathological love of proof.[7]

In the social sciences this idea is sometimes expressed as Campbell's law.[8]

> The more any quantitative social indicator is used for social decision-making, the more subject it will be to corruption pressures and the more apt it will be to distort and corrupt the social processes it is intended to monitor.

DOCTOR'S HEALTH

I was ill once. I asked my registrar's advice. He took one look at me and said, 'Bad luck, Peter. Remember that if you die we'll send Michelle a nice bunch of flowers . . . and then get on with our own lives.' He was right.

A Scottish patient gave me the Lanarkshire classic: 'There's nae pockets in a shrood!'

There is an old saying, 'a doctor who treats himself has a fool for a patient'. We judge other people's symptoms reasonably well, but when we are the patient we tend to be either oversensitive (and thereby neurotic) or overspecific (and thereby delay getting treatment until far too obviously ill). An ill doctor has impaired judgement and concentration and is a risk to himself and maybe to his or her patients. Sadly, too many medico-legal problems and GMC cases have occurred in doctors who had not got illness treated well – often because they had not presented in the first place.

Your illness is a personal tragedy. I hope you get it treated well. Causing harm to patients as a result of it is not excusable.

Look after your own health and sanity first. Your greatest gift to your patients is a healthy and intelligent you.

SOME POINTS ON HEALTH

In my article 'Between health and illness'[9] I suggest that health is best seen as an ongoing outcome from the continuing processes of living life well. 'Living life well' would be defined in terms of wealth, relationships, coherence, fitness, and adaptability, with disease avoidance playing only a minor part.

It is worthwhile having a positive definition of health. For day-to-day medicine the 'absence of disease' is often helpful, but it is not really an adequate concept for full health. Health is often conceived in negative terms, as something lost, or something to be regained. The more positive views of health see it as a form of capacity for action. Mildred Blaxter describes the balance of views well in her book *Health*.[10]

The summary points are as follows:

- The presence of a disease does not necessarily render an individual unhealthy.
- A medical cure can only take an individual back to where they were before the illness; it is unlikely to render them better in either a physiological or a moral way.
- The justification for accepting medical treatment is that the alternative is worse.
- Being 'not ill' does not equate to being healthy.
- Being 'not healthy' does not equate to being ill, nor to the presence of disease.
- There is a distinction to be drawn between remedial and generative mechanisms.
- Treatment of illness, even when successful at arresting the progress of pathology, does not necessarily lead to recovery of health.
- Health is rarely appreciated fully as itself – is more often reflected by its loss or absence.
- Good health is not in any sense a 'normal' or 'natural' state for any organism.
- There is no moral right to health.
- There is a case for there being a moral right to medical treatment based on the Judaeo-Christian injunction to care for those who are ill.
- The presence of a medical care system may increase a society's sense of coherence and thereby be salutogenic.

One-sentence summary of this section: 'health is best seen as an ongoing outcome from the continuing processes of living life well'.[9]

THE RESILIENCY ADVANTAGE

Over the last 40 years in medicine we have moved towards treating risk factors for illness as diseases in their own right. This may be justified or not but it has some unfortunate consequences.

In physical medicine the prevalence of 'high cardiovascular risk' is 100% in men over the age of 50. If I believe the latest risk tables, on my 50th birthday (3 years away) I should start on aspirin and simvastatin, whatever my then state of measurable health. My cardiovascular risk would already be over 20% over 10 years, and according to recommendations I should accept intervention at this threshold. Personally, I am not sure I like this thought.

In psychological medicine we have majored on the concept of stress and vulnerability. We have slowly moved to where stress is seen as being dangerous and a problem in itself. Al Siebert, in his book *The Resiliency Advantage*,[11] gives the lie to such defeatist thinking. He points out that most humans adapt to stress rather well, and find ways of coping with all sorts of problems. The presence of stress is acknowledged, but as a challenge to deal with, not as a reason for people to crumple. The people in our consulting rooms are the ones in whom the stress-deflecting mechanisms have broken down.

When you see a patient who is under 'stress' get lots of detail about the context, what it is that they specifically cannot cope with, and examples of other things they have handled well in the past. Then ask them what strategies they used to handle the problem then and whether they can use them again in the new situation. Often they can.

Try not to turn stress into the medical illness depression.

Stress is a part of life and most humans handle it very well themselves. Sometimes they need a hand from others. Sometimes they just need a little nudge out from whatever rut they have got themselves into. As one (as far as I know unnamed) doctor put it, 'Life is rather like a cesspool. Sometimes our job is to get people down to the shallower end.'

Turning all the stresses and strains of life, whether physiological or psychological, into diseases is not good medicine for reasons Dr Iona Heath (among others) regularly explains.

Humans are surprisingly resilient creatures, and the more we can bolster one another's resilience, the better.

A MNEMONIC TO HELP WITH PROBLEM-SOLVING

I always attribute this summary to Dr Seth Jenkinson, but he says he borrowed it from someone else, although he cannot remember who. It is a useful map of techniques open to us for problem-solving.

Any problem can be solved by one of the following strategies:

- denial
- sort out the problem
- sort out how you respond to the problem
- move away from the problem.

Denial is everyone's favourite first answer. Remember Sir Humphrey Appleby's (from the BBC television series *Yes Minister*) maxim of never to believe anything until it has been denied at least twice. It is the 'don't think of a pink elephant' symptom. Does anyone ever give a vote of confidence to Sir Alex Ferguson? Does anyone deny a problem that doesn't exist? If it should go without saying, why is someone saying it now? Denial is annoying when you encounter it, and funny when it breaks down. Keeping a straight face when it breaks down, and resisting the temptation to say 'I told you so' is sometimes helpful.

Sorting out the problem is often difficult, and it may take more resource and energy than you personally can muster. It may take many meetings.

Sorting out how you respond to the problem is very powerful, but it often takes us all a while to 'get our heads around things'.

Moving away from a problem is sometimes expedient, especially if a situation carries danger in it. Working in a poor practice is an example of where this may become necessary. The battered wife fleeing her husband is another – this strategy works well for immediate safety. However, if you keep on moving each time a problem arises, eventually you have to start thinking about yourself. What weather do you always take around with you?

PARKINSON'S LAW

Parkinson's law states: 'Work expands so as to fill the time available for its completion.'[12] This has been observed in many settings. For readers it may work better as the realisation that if you set time boundaries, work will stay within them. If you do not, then you will be the last one out of the building each night. If that happens you are not working harder than your colleagues, you are just less efficient.

CAMPBELL'S LAW

This is a very useful observation from Dr Bill Campbell, one of the GPs in my training practice in Strathaven.[8] It goes, **'One o'clock is lunchtime. Only break this rule if someone is dying.'** This has been a key part of my staying sane as a GP.

Anyone organising lunchtime meetings and not providing lunch, or at the very least allowing people to bring in their own, is inhospitable.

HUTBER'S LAW

Hutber's law states that 'improvement means deterioration'. It is a somewhat cynical but often, sadly, accurate observation by author and economist Patrick Hutber about the difference between 'a change' and 'an improvement'. The two are not necessarily synonymous, however much people trying to sell you a view or a product might wish it to be so. The medical version of it could be the old surgical joke, **'the operation was a great success, but sadly the patient died'**.

THE GOLDEN MEAN

Aristotle described the idea of the golden mean.[13] Basically, for any virtue there are two vices: one, its excess and the other, its lack. For example, in medicine there is a spectrum between the hyperactive activity of *furor therapeuticus*, with its attendant over-investigation and overtreatment of patients, and the languid and lamentable lack of urgency and curiosity that can be seen in some doctors. Somewhere between these two extremes lies a golden mean of sensible curiosity, balanced treatment and sufficient intervention to meet the need. Younger doctors tend towards *furor therapeuticus*, as they have newly discovered knowledge and skills and are keen to try them out. Older doctors tend to have spent their early excess energy; however, they need to be careful that they do not run out of curiosity and energy completely.

Other examples of spectra between excess and lack are rashness-courage-cowardice, vulgarity-magnificence-pettiness, vanity-magnanimity-pusillanimity. In physiology we could have pathogenesis-homeostasis-salutogenesis. It is important to note that the exact balance between a virtue and its two vices shifts continuously, and it has to be struck sensibly in a particular situation.

Aristotle maintained the golden mean did not apply for some emotions and actions (e.g. murder), as some things are always wrong.

GET A NOTE FROM YOUR DOCTOR: THE GANFYD SYNDROME

Adrian Kenny introduced me to the acronym GANFYD, and I can claim some credit for helping to popularise the term via Doctors.net.uk.[14] No, the Ganfyddiau are not a range of mountains in Wales, but GANFYD requests do add to the mountains of paper (or electronic lists of tasks) in GP surgeries. GANFYD requests waste a lot of GP time and GP appointments to no good clinical purpose. The requests are usually initiated by some minor functionary who remains nameless and who believes that a doctor's note will enable them to do something they otherwise could not do for a patient (their client or customer). Such requests are not like proper official requests from named individuals (e.g. a lawyer or a personnel officer) who commission us to write a sensible medical report. Instead, they are requests in which someone somewhere (e.g. the person in the office) has apparently said, 'Get a note from your doctor'. The patient interprets this as an instruction and sets off to see the doctor with a prior expectation already established that such a thing as a 'doctor's note' actually exists and that the doctor will just write it for them. They are then disappointed when either you decline or you agree to write it but for a fee.

My recommended approach is to write a letter (aka a GANFYD Deflector Shield) that helps you get out of such requests firmly and politely. The basic rule is that you do not provide anything by way of a report when you do not know what you are being asked for or the person to whom you are writing. You can bend over backwards trying to write down all the correct details to convey the requested message by your messenger patient . . . then often you find the organisation never wanted a report in the first place!

Dear Sir/Madam

Request for a medical report/doctor's certificate

I have been told by my patient .... that your organisation needs me to provide your organisation with a medical report/certificate regarding:

....

Please note: I can only legally provide a report/certificate if regulations such as the Access to Medical Reports Act 1988 have been complied with. Providing a medical report/certificate for other agencies in this situation is not an NHS responsibility and is therefore not funded by the NHS. If your organisation requires a medical report/certificate the costs of providing such a report or certificate is the responsibility of your agency making the request and not your client/my patient. My fee for this report will be £xx and this needs to be paid in advance.

   If your organisation does require a medical report or certificate in order to make your decision accurately then you should:
a. obtain signed consent from the patient for release of medical information
b. write to the relevant doctor detailing such information you may require
c. send the appropriate fee.

If you are not prepared to go through this proper process I regret I am unable to provide my professional opinion.

Yours sincerely,

Dr Sensible Report Writer

Date...........................

REFERENCES

1 Starfield B, Shi L, Macinko J. Contribution of primary care to health systems and health. *Milbank Q.* 2005; **83**(3): 457–502.

2 Antonovsky A. *Unravelling the Mystery of Health: how people manage stress and stay well.* San Francisco: Jossey-Bass; 1987.

3 Rose G. Sick individuals and sick populations. *Int J Epidemiol.* 1985; **14**(1): 32–8.

4 Koch R. *The 80/20 Principle: the secret of achieving more with less.* London: Nicholas Brealey; 1998.

5 Covey S. *The Seven Habits of Highly Effective People.* 15th anniversary ed (2004). New York: Simon & Schuster; 1989.

6 Goodhart CAE. Monetary relationships: a view from Threadneedle Street. *Papers in Monetary Economics.* Reserve Bank of Australia; 1975.

7 Kenny A, Davies P. *Probophilia – a disease of our time.* Civitas: The Institute for the Study of Civil Society. Available at: www.civitas.org.uk/nhs/download/probophilia. pdf (accessed 9 March 2012).

8 Campbell D. *Assessing the Impact of Planned Social Change.* Hanover, NH: The Public Affairs Center, Dartmouth College; 1976. Available at: www.eric.ed.gov/ PDFS/ED303512.pdf (accessed 9 March 2012).

9 Davies P. Between health and illness. *Perspect Biol Med.* 2007; **50**(3): 444–52.

10 Blaxter M. *Health.* Cambridge: Polity Press; 2004.

11 Siebert A. *The Resiliency Advantage.* San Fransisco: Berrett-Koehler; 2005.

12 Parkinson CN. Parkinson's law. *Economist.* 19 November 1955.

13 Aristotle. *Ethics.* JAK Thompson, trans. London: Penguin Classics; 1953.

14 Ganfyd. *Get a Note from Your Doctor.* Available at: www.ganfyd.org/index. php?title=Get_a_note_from_your_doctor (accessed 17 December 2011).

FURTHER READING

- Antonovsky A. *Health, Stress and Coping.* San Francisco: Jossey-Bass; 1979.
- Davies P. Between health and illness. *Perspect Biol Med.* 2007; **50**(3): 444–52.
- Davies P, Jenkinson S. Interpreting the evidence. *Student BMJ.* 2008; **16**: S26–7.
- Garbutt G, Davies P. Should the practice of medicine be a deontological or utilitarian enterprise? *J Med Ethics.* 2011; **37**(5): 267–70.
- Magee B. *The Story of Philosophy.* London: Dorling-Kindersley; 1998.
- Westin S, Heath I. Thresholds for normal blood pressure and serum cholesterol. *BMJ.* 2005; **330**(7506): 1461–2.

Chapter 20

Ongoing learning and support: what's the best way to achieve this?

Peter Davies and Lindsay Moran

Ars longa, vita brevis, occasio praeceps, experimentum periculosum, iudicium difficile. (The art is long, life is short, opportunity fleeting, experiment dangerous, judgement difficult.)

—Hippocrates

To laugh often and much; to win the respect of intelligent people and the affection of children ... to leave the world a better place ... to know even one life has breathed easier because you have lived. This is to have succeeded.

—Ralph Waldo Emerson

Young GPs make an abrupt transition from the cosiness of their vocational training scheme (VTS) into a rough world of general practice. They do not always understand fully what they have let themselves in for. They do not always understand fully the world they are encountering. As Hippocrates points out, the art of medicine is long, life is short and it takes time and risk to get it right.

We hope that by the end of this book you are now a lot more clued up about what is going on, and to the opportunities open to you as a new GP. We also hope you are a bit wiser about some of the difficulties and threats you may encounter and that you now have some strategies in place to keep you away from them.

In this final chapter we hope to show you some ways in which you can continue your exploration of life and work safely, providing yourself with additional support and opportunity to encounter new ideas and learning. Our basic belief is that enjoyment and interest of life is in direct proportion to the number of interesting people you can meet and make decent relationships with. **Our strength and our capacity for action lies in our relationships.**

Friendships formed on the VTS are often enduring. Some VTS groups form themselves into ongoing groups that used to be called 'young principals groups'. You knew it was time to wind them up when the first young principal in the group reached their 50th birthday. These days some such groups still flourish under various names. If there is one near you it may well be worth joining. Alternatively, get a group of you together and set up your own. These groups are particularly useful in the first few years after you leave VTS and while you are getting yourself established.

Some sessional GP groups are forming and these can be very useful for sessional and locum doctors. Sometimes 'locum chambers' have a continuing professional development programme as part of their terms of membership.

Some practices are very supportive and will do much to help you settle in. They are unlikely to provide much ongoing reflection and development but at least they will look after you well as you do the work.

Some GPs just power their way through life and the profession, with no obvious external need for support. They may be very internally referenced, or more likely they draw their support from somewhere, and it is not obvious to others where this is.

Some GPs get their support from outside groups – maybe a walking club, a cycling club, a church, mosque or similar.

For young female GPs with children, the myriad antenatal, postnatal, breast-feeding, mothers and toddlers groups and so on are a superb resource. Even as a dad I have enjoyed going to some of these.

Some GPs get their support from family members, although this is not always the best, as they may not fully understand your exact professional strains, and your web of relationships with family is likely to be tangled enough already.

When I was a young GP I found meeting the other doctors in the area via East Kilbride Doctors on Call service was a good way of learning from other people. Out-of-hours service providers can still be a good place to meet a varied selection of colleagues from across an area.

Some groups meet online, and the fora at Doctors.net.uk will soon provide you with many colleagues across the UK. Some groups have private membership online sites, e.g. the Google group for Yorkshire First5® (https://groups.google.com/forum/?fromgroups#!forum/yorkshire-rcgp-first5). The online world has its perils – it is all recorded, and you may not know exactly whom you are talking with.

I think the key point that comes out of all this is that, **as a doctor, you need**

some sort of support system in place for your professional self. Ideally it will be based on reciprocation and mutual self-help. **We should be looking after one another, sometimes giving help, and sometimes receiving it**.

Now having got support needs out of the way, we need to think about who we allow to influence and shape your career. Who will you choose to follow and learn from? Who will you take instruction from? Who will help you to raise your performance level a notch or two? Who will you turn to for help with career progression?

Of course the answer to such questions depends on who you are and what your aspirations are. If I can give you any hint on this it is only to take advice about your work and how to improve it from someone with expertise in your own field, or with significant expertise in a different field of equivalent standing to your own. Many people offer help and advice, and with good intentions. You need to be adept and active in selecting the people you allow to bring their influence into your life.

As you progress through your career you will realise that you have two groups of skills: your **specific craft knowledge** of medicine and your more **generic knowledge** of communication patterns, influence, how to implement changes and so forth. However much our specific craft and specialty knowledge diverges in the early years after medical qualification, when you look at high performance in many fields – both across medical specialties and across professions – later in life you will find that **the leadership and influence skills show remarkable convergence**. However, one thing most leaders in a field have to have is decent craft knowledge as a basic starting point. Without this basic ability in place you lack credibility with the people performing the work. For example, although a lawyer and a doctor could swap notes and learn a lot from each other, a doctor would not be a credible partner in a law firm, nor would a lawyer be a credible partner in a doctor's surgery. Yet many of the problems they face at the organisational level would be quite similar in nature (e.g. how to motivate the staff). I suspect the characteristics of a good senior partner in a law firm would be very similar to those of a good senior partner in a GP practice.

One quick way of learning things is to learn from role models, both the good examples and the dire warnings you have met over time. We turn to these next.

GOOD EXAMPLES, DIRE WARNINGS AND MAKING YOUR WAY IN BETWEEN

We all have certain people whom we regard highly and certain people whom we regard less well. We have people whom we regard as good examples of the kind of thought, behaviour and action we want to emulate. We have other people who teach us exactly the kind of thought, behaviour and actions we wish to avoid.

How can we work out which person belongs to which group for us? How can we go from our immediate emotional reactions to working out exactly what it is that we want to emulate or avoid? How can we work out criteria for good examples and dire warnings? And how can we make them specific enough to be useful, and not so general that we write someone off unfairly over one minor lapse in behaviour?

We are here basically in the territory of how we learn from others.

One technique I can recommend is a '**wall of gratitude**'. This is a list or maybe a picture board of people who have taught you something. We are none of us self-made: we are all the product of many interactions over time. Who would you put on your wall of gratitude? The suggestion is to name the people and write a brief statement about what exactly you learned from each one of them.

I can think of many, many people who have helped me over time. A little bit here, another bit there, gradually a synthesis emerges that is part me and part others. For example, I am always grateful to a cardiology registrar who discussed heart failure care with me and said, 'Yes, they do die, don't they?' This was just what I needed to hear at the time he said it, and it allowed me to relax about managing such patients and to accept that some of them would die, that it was just the nature of the illness and not a failure of my medicine.

There are many others who have helped my development over time and to whom I am grateful. I cannot pay them back, but what I can do is to pass on what I have learned to others coming up behind me. This obeys the Hippocratic injunction to teach the sons of those who taught me – the constant need for us to help those coming after us to grow strongly themselves.

You can view this development along a **spectrum of dependence, independence and interdependence**.

When we are young we are entirely dependent on our parents. We had no option but to hope and trust that our parents were right – indeed, the idea they may at times be wrong probably does not emerge at this stage.

As we progress through our teenage years and our early twenties, we (at least I hope we do) begin to think for ourselves. We begin to question, and later still we learn how to question properly and to a point, not just as an end in its stroppy self. By about the age of 25 we tend to be quite independent characters.

Later, we begin to form our adult relationships – marriage, profession, career and so forth – and we begin to realise that we are a part within a whole, and that others know rather a lot that we do not and that we can learn from their experience. Indeed, we start to move away from notions of ourselves as some sort of 'superman', or 'the therapeutic thunderbolt' or 'the only person who's ever noticed this problem' and instead move towards thinking, 'I hope I am playing my part well in all this. I hope I am adding something to the whole.' At this stage we move more to networked relationships and to selecting which causes are worth pursuing and which are better left alone or to others. We start to accept direction from sensible others (e.g. local medical committee chairs) and accepting their hints when they say, 'There's a problem over there you could help us with.' We start to build up a 'mastermind group' of helpful others whom we can contact for their wisdom.

DIRE WARNINGS

We will all have seen some people or colleagues who by their thoughts, behaviours and actions fill us with dread or revulsion. It is well worth recalling such people to mind periodically, and working out exactly why they appeared so dire to you. Learn what you can from them, and then apply some compassion to them. I'll show you why shortly. Even as you recall their badness, be grateful for the lesson they have taught you – even if it isn't the one they had meant to give you.

Remember that we are each doing the best we can with the knowledge and materials we have to hand. Many doctors are competitive and motivated powerfully by a fear of failure. This is a powerful and unbalanced drive, and can lead to competitive and unbalanced behaviour. It often leads to great success, but with a restless inability to enjoy what one has achieved. Often arrogance is a cover for fear. The angry, roaring surgeon who has terrified his operating theatre staff is brought down to earth as the sister gives the message, suspiciously well timed to coincide perfectly with the crux of the operation, 'Mrs Cutfaster has just rung and asked you to bring two pints of milk and a dozen eggs home with you tonight.' She then adds, 'You won't forget this time, will you?'

Fear makes us do many silly things, and in medicine the fears of the patients are often equalled by the fears of the doctor. 'What have I got?' is matched by 'Will I be able to handle this?' The fear on both the side of the patient and the side of the doctor is of being overwhelmed by events – either their number or their severity.

Macbeth's comment, 'Come what come may. Time and the hour runs through the roughest day' is a consoling thought when things seem to be getting on top of you.

SOME COMPASSION

Marshall Goldsmith is a US business consultant and author of an excellent book on 360° appraisals entitled *What Got You Here Won't Get You There.*[1] The book's key point is that most of us have progressed to where we have got to today partly because of our great intelligence and many good qualities and partly because many people have been kind enough to celebrate these and look away from the less appealing sides and aspects of ourselves. Goldsmith is an executive coach, usually helping companies with the ranks just below chief executive officer and senior directors. He works with this next stratum of senior managers by using

360° feedback to help them to get the rough edges off their behaviour and character, helping them to safely progress up to chief executive officer and similar very
senior positions. If the rough edges and character flaws had gone unchecked, the
risk was of a very capable chief executive officer destroying a company because
of one minor character flaw. The minor flaw would be tolerable at lower levels,
but when exposed to widespread view at senior levels could be disastrous.

Perhaps to some extent we are all always simultaneously good examples and
dire warnings to others. Be aware that what we recognise and criticise in others
may well be things we would rather not have within ourselves.

Our ability to pick out flaws on others is rarely matched by our ability to spot
our own flaws. The Reverend Eli Jenkins in Dylan Thomas's play *Under Milk
Wood*[2] is worth recalling here. After a play full of carping and criticism of each
character by the others, he comes out with the great prayer:

> We are not wholly bad or good
> Who live our lives under Milk Wood,
> And Thou, I know, wilt be the first
> To see our best side, not our worst.

Let's hope most of us decide to see the better side rather than the worse side of
one another.

MENTORING, COACHING AND SIMILAR ACTIVITIES

Is external support for your professional role and development useful? We are all
familiar with the idea of a sporting coach and the processes they use to improve
achievement in the sporting arena. In recent years we have seen the development
of coaching and mentoring as means to improve work and intellectual performance in the work arena. Does this process work? If so, who should you get to do
it for you? I don't think there is a definitive answer to such questions yet.

Some doctors are lucky enough to get informal mentoring – a benign senior
partner, or another helpful older colleague basically does it for them. As an
example, I learned plenty discussing various ideas with Dr Seth Jenkinson when
I moved to work with him in Mixenden in 2001. Our discussions worked and
generated many ideas and papers and have helped me with much of my subsequent successes. The account of the Rose paradox in Chapter 19 is largely based
on my discussions with Seth. Seth was the kind of colleague who just lobbed
such ideas into a conversation.

Sometimes an external coach is useful. I think it's useful when you need an
external perspective on your work, someone who is not currently entangled
with your concerns and processes. Although such a detached viewpoint is useful, the coach is relying entirely on your account of reality and of course won't

get the picture filled in by meeting the other players in the drama of your life. The coach will, however, help you to clarify your account and thinking and also to question your assumptions about why others are acting as they do and are. Such a coach can be a great sounding board and may help you significantly sort your thinking so your stress levels reduce, so your effectiveness rises. As with all these enterprises the more material you contribute to the process, the more you reflect on it and reframe it, the more you get out of it. To some extent the coach or mentor is there to help you bring out whatever is already within you, just a bit more quickly than you would manage to do yourself.

The key to any such relationship is that the mentor and mentee trust each other and work well together.

Such a service is very helpful to some people and not others. If you are thinking about it, it is worth a try, and it may well prove very helpful to you.

Some sort of trial, and review after a period is sensible. Unlike training or appraising there are no formal qualifications in mentoring and coaching. Although most people who set themselves up in such roles are well trained and there are various respected training centres, there are no guarantees. You'll need to do a bit of research to decide if you can trust the person or not.

Appraisal is not mentoring. Some skills are common between the two activities, but as appraisal is currently set up it is an annual event, whereas mentoring is an ongoing process. Appraisal has a set of specific requirements, whereas mentoring will work with whatever material is currently relevant to the person being mentored. Whether appraisal would be better adapted towards a mentoring role is debatable and there are no current plans or funding towards making any such move.

Sometimes a mentor may be a useful answer and follow-up for some problems identified at appraisal.

FELLOWSHIP

As you progress in the profession after 5 years of continuous membership of the college you become eligible to be considered for fellowship. To me, fellowship is about belonging and contribution to our specialty. It is awarded as recognition of contribution and effort to the work of general practice in the consulting room and in other areas of activity such as education, research and leadership. Currently fellowship is too specific – only about 10% of GPs have it. They all deserve it. There are many others out there who are very good GPs and who are making huge contributions to their practices and areas but who have not got the recognition that fellowship bestows – a recognition they would richly deserve.

Fellowship is a very enjoyable mid-career boost for GPs, and it reaffirms and values your contribution to your patients and your profession. There is a one-off cost to fellowship in the RCGP. In other specialties the fellowship is paid for by subsequent increased subscriptions. For new GPs it is worth thinking about when you will upgrade your membership to fellowship.

CONCLUSION

However you approach general practice and whatever level of effectiveness you work at, you will be doing useful and valuable work. UK-based doctors with MRCGP are in demand, in classic general practice roles and beyond. We are wanted both in the UK and abroad. Although you are well trained now, you will enjoy your career more if you retain a relentless curiosity and fascination with life and medicine and if you continually keep learning – about medicine, about leadership and about life in general.

> In a time of drastic change it is the learners who inherit the future. The learned usually find themselves equipped to live in a world that no longer exists.[3]

Eric Hoffer's quote above sums up where we are at present. When have we ever lived in times that are not changing?

The authors of this book hope that this book has equipped you with useful extra knowledge to adapt what you have learned already into the actual world of British general practice. We hope that you will have an enjoyable and prosperous career and that you will do well for your patients, your colleagues and yourself. We hope that, in whatever way, you will make a valuable contribution to general practice and primary care.

We wish you all the best for your future.

REFERENCES

1 Goldsmith M, Reiter M. *What Got You Here Won't Get You There: how successful people become even more successful!* London: Profile; 2008.
2 Thomas D. *Under Milk Wood: a play for voices.* Dent; 1954.
3 Hoffer E. *Reflections on the Human Condition.* London: Millington; 1974.

Index

80/20 rule (Pareto principle) 206–7

accountants
    and GP partnerships 53, 57, 174
    and locum work 63–4
action, spheres of 106
administration
    in GP partnerships 52
    and locum work 63–5
AiT (Associates in Training) committee 3
alcohol addiction 148
anonymity, collusion of 62, 171
APMS (alternative provider medical
    services) 175–7
appraisal
    complaints and compliments in
        99–100, 188
    feedback in 97–8
    first 100–1, 201
    forms for 94–6
    and freelance work 62
    key points on 76, 92–3
    and mentoring 221
    preparation for 93–4, 101–2
    and revalidation 109
    toolkits for 87, 101
    weaknesses of system 102–3
armed forces 33

Bevan, Aneurin 22, 125–6
BMJ (British Medical Journal) 84, 87
British Medical Association (BMA), GPs
    Committee 21
business development managers 181–2

Calderdale
    commissioning in 31
    GPwSIs in 30
Campbell's law 211

capacity assessments 33–4
cause for concern investigations 111
CCGs (clinical commissioning groups)
    and primary care 133–4
    vacancies in 120–1
    value of 130–1
change, resistance to 39–40
Churchill, Winston 46, 115–16
clinical audit
    in appraisal 93, 96
    as CPD 85
    and plaudit 188–9
clinical governance
    and appraisal 103
    channels of 110–12
    importance of 77
    and licence to practice 80
    and revalidation 107–8
clinical negligence 192
coaching 220–1
cognitive dissonance 117–18
coherence 155, 204–5, 209
College of General Practitioners, see RCGP
commissioning
    description of 126–7
    need for 127–30
    role of in GP work 30–1, 131
    whole-system 134
commissioning consortia 9, 31, 41
commissioning support organisations 131
communication breakdowns 185
communication skills 165, 171–2, 186, 188,
    193
compassion 219–20
competence, ladder of 83
complaints
    in appraisal 99
    dealing with 183–5, 193
    learning from 187–8

223

complaints (*continued*)
  replying to 185–6
  roles in 189–91
  types of 185
consultation skills 2, 122, 167–9
consultations
  fundamental importance of 37–8
  overcrowded 166, 169–71
  threats to 167–8
  in work of GPs 29–30
CPD (continuing professional
  development)
  and appraisal 82, 84, 86, 102–3
  and complaints 99
  in First5® 4
  groups for 89–91
  importance of 82–3
  and licence to practice 80–1
  for locums 66, 216
  measuring 85–6
  methods of 87–9
  for new GPs 54
  recording 86–7, 93–4, 96
  reflecting on 84
  for salaried GPs 71, 73
curiosity 84–5, 163, 222
CV (curriculum vitae) 47–51, 63

denial 148, 151, 210–11
depression 76, 148, 161, 210
DH (Department of Health)
  on commissioning 126
  input from doctors 43
  medical advice for 33
  role of 127
doctor shopping 197
doctor's bag 143–5
drugs, controlled 145
duty doctors 141

e-learning 88
economists, attitudes to professionals 8–9
emotions 149, 183–5, 196
enhanced services 30, 176, 178
ePortfolio 20, 86–7, 201
experience, gaining 199–200
expert witnesses 33, 193

failure, fear of 219
fellowship 19, 221–2

First5®
  birth of 2–4
  and GMS contracts 43
  and mentoring 200
  on Twitter 89
followership 114–17, 122, 135
foundation trusts 128
freelance work, *see* locum work

GANFYD syndrome, *see* sick notes
gatekeeping 17, 163
General Medical Services contract, *see*
  GMS
general practice, *see* primary care
general practitioners, *see* GPs
General Practitioners Committee 20–1, 42,
  206
global sum 176
GMC (General Medical Council)
  appraisal headings 95–7
  complaints to 186–7
  and doctors' illness 148–9
  and professional regulation 110
  and revalidation 76–8, 107–8
GMS (General Medical Services), use of
  term 175
GMS (General Medical Services) contracts
  and employment for new GPs 43,
    54–5
  health promotion in 21
  and time pressure 166–7
golden mean 212
Goodhart's law 207–8
GP contracts 21, 43, 54, 71
GP partnerships
  benefits and drawbacks of 45, 54–8
  cash flow in 174–5
  cost management in 128–9, 179–81
  dynamics of 38–40
  future of 134, 182
  goal-setting for 105–6
  income streams for 177–9
  insurance for 180
  and locums 60
  management of 181–2
  performance data for 52
  remuneration in 174
  structure and function of 23
GP registrars 2, 20, 175
GP trainers 41, 158

GPs (general practitioners)
    career paths of 135
    effectiveness of 204–5
    as entrepreneurs 61
    essential items for 143–4
    evolution of role in UK 16–18
    health of 147–50, 154–6, 208
    jobs market for 1–2, 54–5
    negative examples of 219
    and NHS 25
    pathology knowledge of 161
    popularity of 204
    private work for 34
    as professionals 7–8
    reports on quality of 11
    roles for 29–35, 40
    support systems for 216–19
    terms of service 206
    training of 19–20
    typical work of 139–41
    variability among 129
GPwSI (GP with a special interest) 30, 34, 53
gratitude, wall of 218

health, positive definition of 208–9
health insurance, history of in UK 16
health screening 32
healthcare
    funding of 24, 127–8
    market in 9
home visits 65, 143–4, 146
homelessness 32
hospital admissions 158–9, 203
humour, sense of 155
Hutber's law 211

ignorance, acknowledging 161
illness
    assessing severity 157–9
    difficult 160–1
income protection insurance 64
information asymmetry 9–10
inverse care law 18

jobs
    finding 45, 47–8
    interviews for 51–3
    nature of 46–7
    preliminary visits to 50–1

Karpman drama triangle 189–91

leadership
    clinical 118–20
    and cognitive dissonance 117–18
    and commissioning 114, 130, 135
    educational 18
    frames of reference 116–17
    qualities of good 115–16
    quotations on 113–14
    skills of 217
    taking on 120–2
learning, from colleagues 88
learning credits 85–6
learning styles 82–3
licence to practice
    and clinical governance 77
    maintaining 80–1, 111–12
    time limit on 107
local medical committees (LMCs) 31, 41–2
local training programmes 41
locum agency 62
locum chambers 63, 216
locum work
    benefits and drawbacks of 59–61
    casualisation of 62
    demand for 31
    finding 62–4
    invoices for 67–8
    rates for 64–6
    requirements for 63
    terms and conditions for 66–7
    typical day of 141–2
Luddites 10

managers, and market mechanisms 9–10
maternity locums 60, 65, 200
medical appraisal system 32
medical defence organisations
    GPs working for 33
    and locum work 64
    and poor feedback 98
medical directors
    and appraisal 32, 94, 99–100
    learning about poor performance 103, 111
medical economics 127
medical ecosystem 41
medical effectiveness, levels of 37–44
medical journalism 33

medical journals 84, 87, 89
medicine, as social science 15
medico-legal work 33
mentoring 3, 92, 199–202, 220–1
military medicine 33
minimum practice income guarantee 176
misconduct, serious professional 108, 110, 187
MRCGP exam
  beginnings of 19
  importance of 20
MSF (multi-source feedback) 93, 97–8, 101

NASGP (National Association of Sessional GPs) 59, 65–6, 68, 89
National Commissioning Board 130–1
National Patient Safety Agency 43, 97
negligence actions 99, 110, 186–7, 192–3
new media 88–9
NHS (National Health Service)
  core income from 177
  economics of 127–8, 173–5
  GPs in 17–18
  pitfalls of 21–4
  at regional level 42
  reorganisation of 24–5
  stress in 153–4
NHS Choices website 47, 52, 63
nMRCGP exam 2–3, 20
nursing homes 32

occupational health 32, 111, 187
out-of-hours care 180

parity system 57
Parkinson's law 211
pathogenesis 150, 154
pathology, detecting 163
patient feedback (PF) 93, 98, 101
Patient Health Questionnaire 117
patient safety 119, 149, 187
Patient Satisfaction Questionnaire 98
Patient Source Feedback (PSF) 97–8
patients
  death of 152–3, 186
  expectations of 170
  heartsink 195–8
  relationship with 188–9

pensions, for locums 64, 68
perfectionism 153
performance management 41, 43, 111
performers list status 103
personal development plans (PDPs) 86, 94, 105–6
PMS (personal medical services) 175, 177
practice managers 181, 185
presenteeism 150
primary care
  business model of 173–4
  effectiveness of 205
  history of in UK 13–17
  and homelessness 32
  NHS priority of 131
  and public health 23, 205–6
  quality of 11, 21
  and secondary care 131–3
  time pressure on 165–6, 170
  training for 19–20
primary care trusts
  and commissioning 128, 130
  and practice contracts 175–6
  vacancies in 120
prisons 32
problem definition 165–6, 172
problem-solving 151–2, 167, 210–11
probophilia 208
professions
  economics of 8–11
  general practice as 16
  nature of 7–8
  and quality control 76–7, 81
public health 16, 23–4, 32, 205

Quality, Innovation, Productivity and Prevention 177
Quality and Outcomes Framework (QOF)
  and GP partners 71
  and health promotion 21
  and Pareto principle 207
  description of 176
  imposed leadership of 117
  income from 177–8
  in job interviews 52–3

RCGP (Royal College of General Practitioners)
  courses for new GPs 87

current role of 20–1
foundation of 2–3, 18–20
and mentoring 200
online resources from 88
RCGP toolkit 86, 102
referees 49
reference, frames of 25, 43, 117, 133
referrals 163, 171, 204
reflection
  in action 100
  on complaints and compliments 99
  evidence of 97–8
reflective commentary 94
rent, notional 57, 176
research
  and appraisal 94, 96
  and leadership 121
  roles in 31
resiliency 209–10
revalidation
  and appraisal 93
  and CPD 78, 82, 84
  and freelance work 62
  preparation for 108–9
  purpose of 76–8, 107–8
  and quality control 32
  requirements for 98
  SEA in 97
  toolkits for 87
RO (responsible officers) 107–9
role models 217–18
Rose paradox 23, 205, 220
Rose question 206
rule of threes 159

salaried GPs
  benefits and drawbacks of 70–2
  earnings of 66, 72–3
  and GP contracts 54–5
  support for 3
  typical day of 142
salary, negotiating 53–4
salutogenesis 154, 204–5, 209, 212

SEA (significant event audit)
  in appraisal 93, 97
  as CPD 85
second opinions 160
self-awareness 219–20
senior partners
  health of 147–8
  leadership role of 38–9, 217
sessional work, *see* locum work
sick notes 16, 212–13
silo thinking 21, 25, 132–3
SMART criteria 105
smartphone apps 145–6
social capital 204–5
social networking 89
strategic health authorities 42
stress
  coping with 149–51, 155
  and leadership 119
  and resiliency 210
  and system inefficiency 133
  and time pressure 167
  types of 152–4
substance misuse services 32
symptom soup 162–4
symptoms, incidence of 162, 203

tax bills 63–4, 68
teaching hospitals 17, 21–2
teaching positions 31, 42
time management 207
Twitter 89

uncertainty, managing 157–64
United States, consultations in 30

vocation 7
VTS (vocational training scheme)
  aftermath of 157, 200, 215
  friendships formed during 216
  limitations of 2

young principals groups 216